MOLLY SHATTUCK

VIBRANT LIVING

21 DAYS to Transform your Body, Burst with Energy, and Live Your Life with Purpose

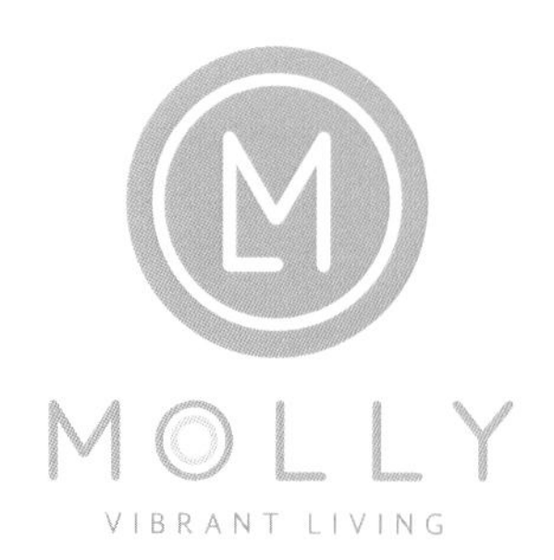
MOLLY
VIBRANT LIVING

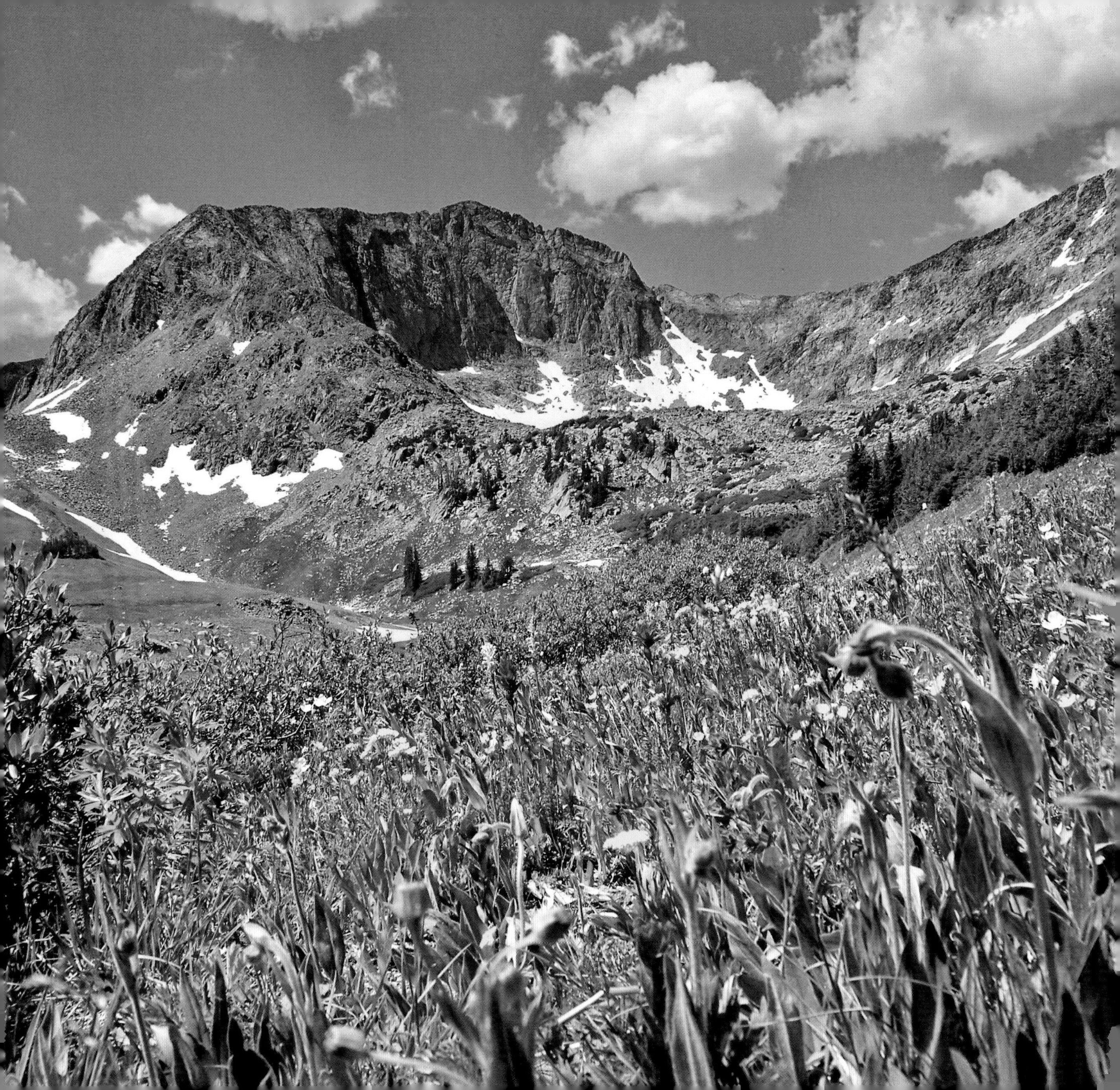

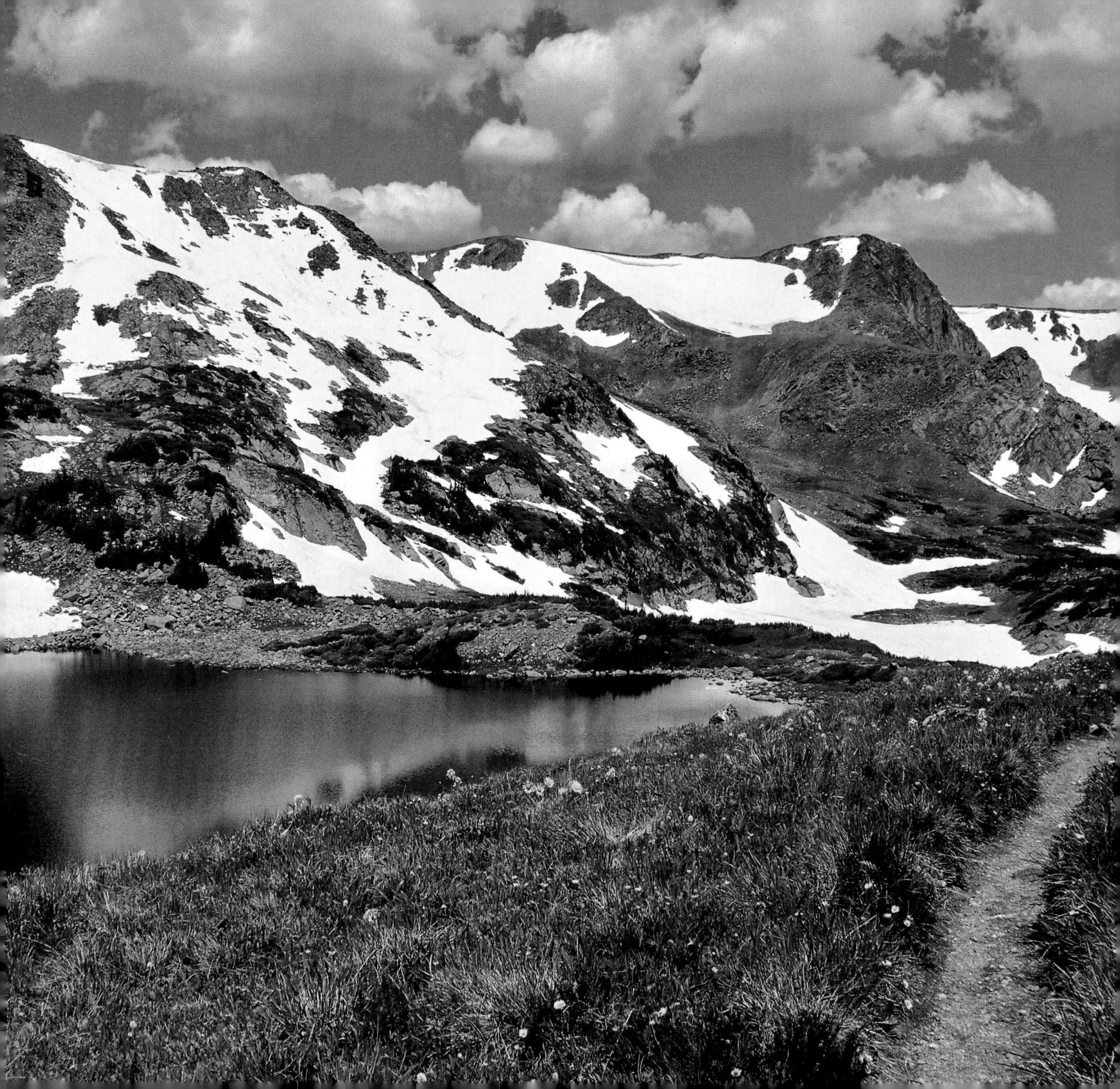

Foreword

Deeply rooted in the value systems of most people are those key elements that create meaning and stability in our lives—a spiritual foundation; sharing a full life with friends and loved ones; making a positive difference in the lives of others; feeling safe both emotionally and financially; and feeling good about ourselves inside and out.

These values are central to our journey through life, yet countless obstacles threaten to derail us from what we value most. One of the most prevalent obstacles is poor health choices. It's fair to say that poor health habits—and the destructive consequences they can leave on our physical and emotional well-being—stop us from living life to the fullest, lead to chronic disease states and cause premature deaths.

Vibrant Living by Molly Shattuck is an inspirational and empowering book aimed at helping all who choose to fully embrace its concepts to improve both their physical and emotional health. Courageously authored from a profound commitment to help, motivate and empower others, Molly's book provides a realistic, back-to-the-basics approach to better health and better habits.

The 21-day program, with its pearls of wisdom thoughtfully interwoven with invigorating physical activities, will work if one truly commits. The journey may not always be easy, but if you put your mind to it—really give yourself to it—*Vibrant Living* will transform your perspective on life. The confidence you gain and the lessons you learn will positively empower you for a lifetime.

Molly's book is unique in that it's not just about taking a pill, being on a quick-results diet, or adhering to demanding strenuous daily exercise. *Vibrant Living* is about lifestyle change, a positive shift in your awareness and understanding of what is really important and what is really doable. What you learn from this book, if adopted, will prove more effective than any medication or diet in terms of making safe and healthy lifestyle choices, achieving lasting weight control, and feeling energetic.

Inspired by courage, truthfulness, a sincere passion for life, and an unyielding dedication to helping others, *Vibrant Living* is a proven road map to excellent health and a full and meaningful life. It will inspire, empower, and arm you with precisely what's needed to live up to the values most important to all human beings.

Let's get started.

Hilton M. Hudson II, M.D., F.A.C.S., F.C.C.P.
Cardiothoracic Surgeon
CEO of HPC, Inc.
Chicago, IL USA

Acknowledgments

Vibrant Living was conceived outdoors, like so many of my grand plans, during a snowshoe adventure in Colorado and my resolve to finish it was strengthened while hiking through the Grand Canyon two months later. Its publication marks another great dream fulfilled, with a virtuous circle of contributors to thank.

I'm grateful to a host of professionals who offered such meaningful counsel. Hilton Hudson, MD, believed in my work and cheered me on to finish it. Roger Blumenthal, MD, took such a personal interest in the book, providing guidance and endorsing me with gusto. Creative book artists John Kudos and Karen Vanderbilt of Studio Kudos made the book as beautiful as the vistas we featured.

I'm thankful to the magnificent state of Colorado for putting on her dazzling best when we shot photos there. Linda and Mitch Hart opened their blooming, brilliant gardens to us, and Vickae Meenach was an angel when we called. Billie and Ross McKnight welcomed us into their waterfall. And Lisa Dennis allowed us to christen her majestic cabin path.

Hearty thanks to a marvelous photography team. Julie Soefer had such a keen eye on location; Harry Dearing III sang and danced day and night and through all the joy that transpired; and the stunning Victoria Calloway brought an expert hand and eye to my face and hair. Samira can now add food and attire stylist to her resume, and she provided an unending source of giggles. Spencer and Wyatt offered assistance in "finding the light" and raised me up as they always do with such pure love. Greg Sileo—friend, photographer and partner for years in serving others in the city of Baltimore—guided me in photo selection and taking last minute shots.

Editing expertise in various stages of the book came from Angela Vennemann, Marlene Rawls and Beth McConnell. Katy Stephens offered her nutritional opinions and put the "jigsaw puzzle" of a bibliography together. And thanks, too, to Jenna Rausch at Hilton Publishing for all the detail work that brought this book to its readership.

Living for others infused this book with meaning. Thank you to Rick Bernstein for the work we do together on the farm and for our rich, higher spirit discussions of connection to the earth and others. Every day, the tireless work of my United Way family—Holly, Elise, Sandy, Mark, Beth, Liz, Amanda, Sheryl, Natalie, Barbara, and Windy—brings hope and healthy food to so many, meeting the basic needs of our community. Skip Howe, your love for educating kids and safe drinking water continues to inspire me.

Business manager Lisa Kraynak brought a great vision to this book and the whole of Molly Vibrant Living. Ashley Greyson of Ribbow Media expertly communicated the book's meaning in Facebook messages and primed the website for community interaction.

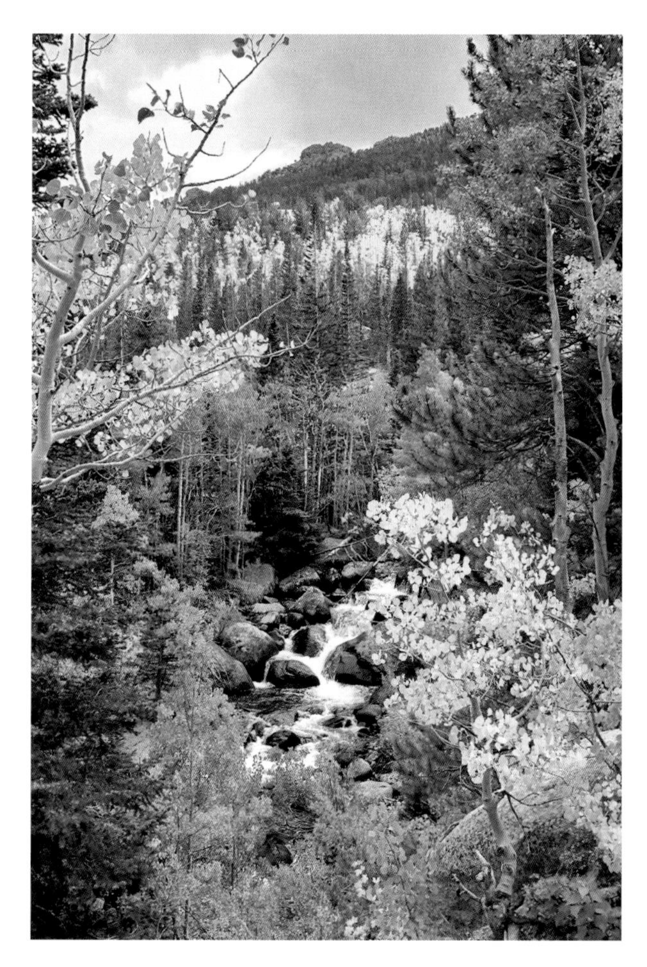

Marg Stark, a woman of faith, an author in her own right and now a dear friend, helped me transform this book into what it is today. She drew out my personal stories and interviewed the clients who share their stories here. Thank you to all the clients who spent 21 days with me, from my days in the beginning to now, especially Karen, Marta, Leslie and Dean who here offer testimonies about their 21-Day Action Plan results. Each of you are dear to me.

Writing this book, I was so often reminded of my beloved friend, Joe Robert, who taught me so much about full-out, courageous and generous living. He was the light shining down on me in Colorado. With me, too, in spirit was my grandmother Lois Mae George, my lifelong role model and the woman who told me I could do anything in life. She is pure faith, hope, love and joy.

Over the years, the Golden Girls—Cheryl, Chrissy, Jen, Joanne, Nicole, Julie, and Babe—have been devoted and loyal, loving friends, readily offering their best beauty pearls for the book. My precious Lillian is a constant source of light and love, even when she was off at play practice during out photo shoot. Stalwart and sweet, Wyatt and Spencer provided me with their expert view on my business, which I will forever value. Mayo lent his continued support, and my sister Lisa George shared her splendid photos throughout this book. My pooch Lizzie Mae enjoyed her time in the spotlight and was my steady companion as I burned the midnight oil—on both the east and west coast time zones—finishing this book.

I am profoundly grateful for the way the Creator moves in my life—giving me calm when clouds roll in, opening my eyes to new possibilities, and connecting me to *real* people who nourish my soul. Ultimately, their energy propels my work, attracting readers like you into our virtuous circle where, together, we can embrace health, give thanks and serve others.

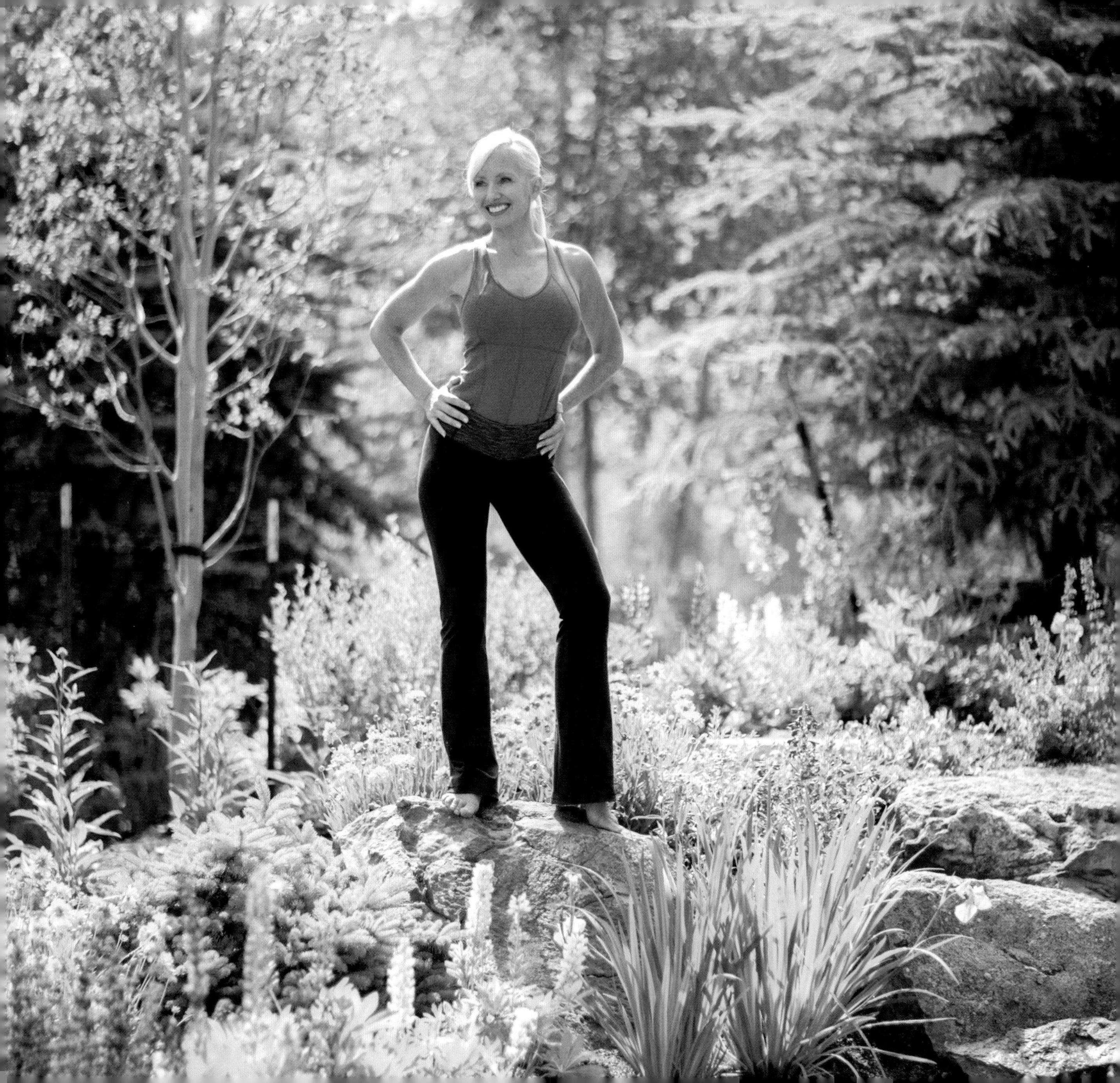

EMBODY YOUR DREAMS

Let's pretend for a moment that tomorrow, there is an open audition being held near you. Or there's a unique opportunity, a splendid new direction for your life.

You would wake up and—boom—this enticing possibility would be within GPS range, bringing a long-held dream into the here and now.

Would you jump out of bed and go?

"The future depends on what you do today."

MAHATMA GANDHI

Picture tomorrow's possibility, big or small. Take a minute or two to allow a few of your fondest life wishes to surface. Maybe you've always wanted to sing the national anthem at a big, public event. Or take salsa lessons with your spouse. Maybe you're interested in devoting a year of your life to a mission—to go to Haiti or the Horn of Africa. Perhaps you want to run a 5K. Keep a gratitude journal. Start your own business. Or take your family on a big vacation.

In Molly Vibrant Living workshops I've led over the past two years, I've interacted with people from all walks of life, in meetings at small and large companies, at churches, universities and women's groups. Among this diverse cross section of the population, a common theme emerged. Less than 1 percent of the participants had identified life dreams. Only a handful had made New Year's resolutions on January 1. Any dream would do—jotted on a napkin or scrawled in an old journal. Yet, in most cases, the people with whom I met had not paused in their busy lives to consider: What would give me greater joy? How might I more passionately employ my God-given gifts? (Throughout this book, when I refer to God, feel free to substitute the word that feels right to you or to your faith experience—be it God, Love, Universe, or the other names you may call a higher power or source of strength and creativity.)

For all of us who get too busy, too enmeshed in today's muck to think about tomorrow's potential, the big break around the corner is likely to pass us by. Life may, accordingly, take on a degree of sameness for days and months and years to come.

So, *what about you?*

Could you muster the courage and the clarity of purpose to go to an audition tomorrow? Would you greet the new day, and this new chance, infused with focus, energy and hope?

TRYOUTS ARE TOMORROW, BRING YOUR BIKINI SHOT

This is what happened to me eight years ago. It had been a lifelong dream of mine to be a NFL cheerleader, and I learned one day in late February that the tryouts for the Baltimore Ravens cheerleading squad were . . . *the very next day*. I was 38 years old, with three children under the age of six, and had spent the better part of the last decade pregnant, nursing and changing diapers. I had not cheered since college. But I still had the itch. Becoming a professional cheerleader had been on "my list" of personal goals since I was 18 years old.

For the audition, I needed a full-body photo of myself in a bikini. Problem was, I didn't own a bikini. So I put on a bra and matching underwear and stood against a plain wall in my bathroom to take the "glam" shot. I showed up at the tryouts the next day in mom-style, knee-length Spandex shorts with a pink top

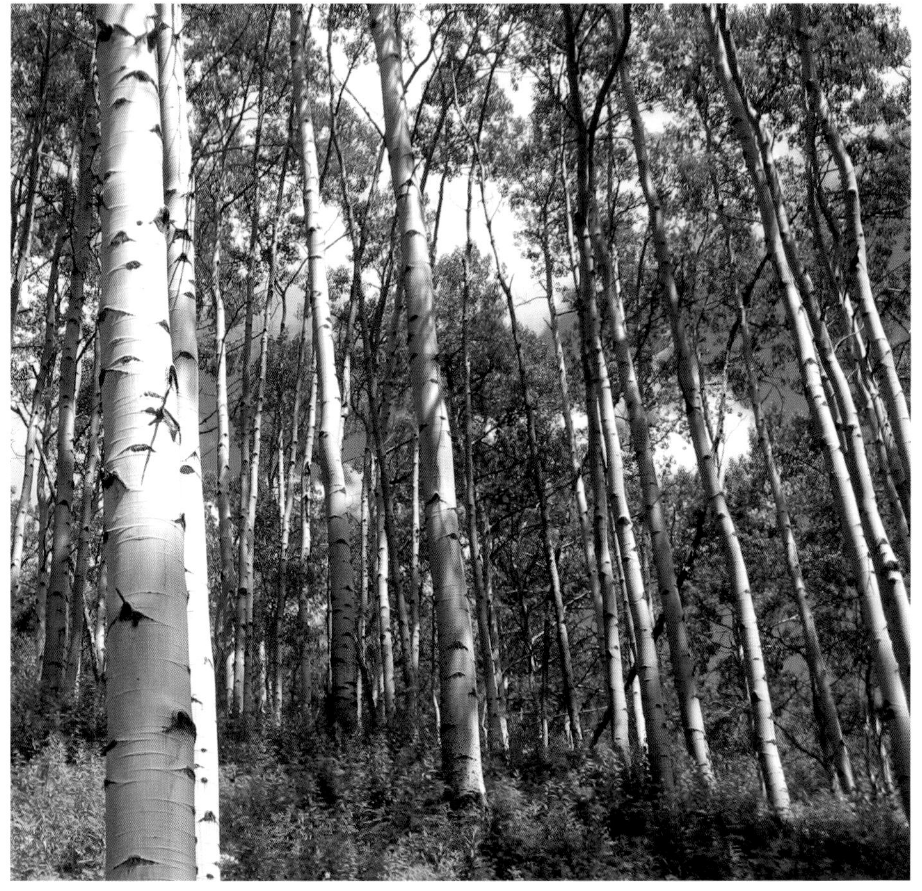

One of my favorite places to be active outside is Colorado, where I have family and friends. The photos we shot for this book were all taken in the central Rocky Mountains.

from Target. It's fair to say I looked a little dated in my attire—among a sea of low-cut sequin tops, booty shorts, big hair and eyelashes.

Four weeks later, after five rounds of cuts, I was named to the squad.

I became, at that time, the oldest cheerleader in NFL history. I cheered for two years on the Baltimore Ravens troop—and served for six more as a part-time coach—with cheerleaders who were, on average, 18 years younger than I was.

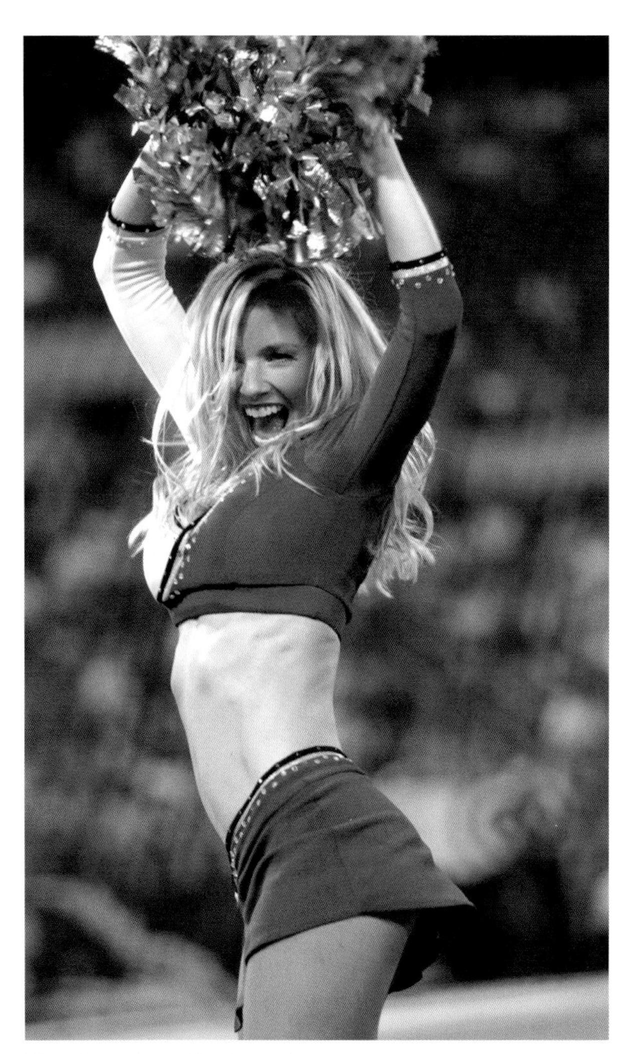

There's nothing like the rush of cheering before a crowd of 70,000 rabid NFL fans! Photo by Napoleon Martinez.

How did I have the *chutzpah* to do it at 38, many asked. First, it never occurred to me that I was too old to do it. Secondly, it was on "my list." Just like climbing Mount Kilimanjaro, the tallest mountain in Africa, was on my list. And running a marathon, all 26.2 miles of it, was on my list.

Truly, my eyes are open all the time to the possibilities around me because I've always maintained a list. And that list becomes the *driving force behind my everyday choices*—the small, seemingly inconsequential daily decisions we make, often without thinking. Like what to eat for lunch and whether we want French fries with that. Or whether we want to work out when we get home from work. Or whether we want to volunteer at our kids' schools or sign up to bring a dish to a homeless shelter.

That's what this book is about: the split-second choices you make every day to fuel your energy or dull it.

To strengthen your body and remain faithful to your life purpose and dreams *or* to make repeated detours of potato chips and weekend-long reality show binges that take you away from the body you want and the life you deserve. After all, neglecting to be intentional—day after day, tiny choice after tiny choice—can lead to a lifetime of poor health, unrealized dreams and lackluster living.

WHAT WOULD YOU DO IF YOU WEREN'T TIRED?

Recently, Sheryl Sandberg, the chief operating officer of Facebook, has asked women the pointed question, what would you do if you weren't afraid? In this book, we ask a related question: *what would you do if you weren't tired?*

What might you accomplish each day if your physical energy was significantly increased? If you were 20, or 50, pounds lighter? If you had more muscle tone and didn't suffer from backaches or knee strain?

What bright ideas or innovations might you usher into the world if your blood sugar didn't rise and fall like a yo-yo all day? How much more playful and loving might you be, as a parent, if stress didn't leave you so frayed?

Just imagine the stereotypes you might consign to the dust bin of history — who says a mom pushing 40 can't be a cheerleader?! — if you could recall precisely what you wanted to say after walking all the way down the hall to say it.

And think how we might all change the world and serve God if our diets really consisted of the bounty of nourishing food we have been given.

OK, take a breath. Because, let's face it, many of us get exhausted *just thinking about* a life of disciplined choices, a life of perpetual, high energy. I get it. I never dreamed before I became a mom that life and its challenges would come *at* me at the pace it does.

From miscarriages to high-risk births, from a broken back to a brain surgery, I've faced my most devastating and glorious moments in the exquisite realm of parenthood. It's not easy to manage the everyday challenges either, as I age and discover my metabolism becomes less forgiving.

Amid these stresses, all of us have quiet moments—on a walk around the neighborhood or perhaps at church on Sunday mornings—when we entertain sweeter possibilities for our lives. When we want *more* for ourselves. And believe we have more to offer God and the world.

Becoming a pom-pom mom, well, it's not everybody's dream. But is your soul tugging on you? Is there something in life you have always wanted to try? Then the **21-Day Action Plan** may help align your habits with the higher purpose to which you are drawn.

WHAT'S THE SECRET?

When you encounter someone with untiring energy, you want to know their secrets. In my hometown of Baltimore, I cart my children to a double-digit array of soccer, football, lacrosse, piano and dance sessions each week. I also lead, help organize or participate in numerous community service projects each year. So I get these questions often:

- Do you *ever* sleep?
- How do you have so much energy?
- How many hours do you work out a day?
- You must never eat dessert, right?
- How do you stay so positive?
- Why do you take that water bottle with you *everywhere*—to every event, even to church?

The truth is, I don't have any secrets. I have never belonged to a gym or hired a personal trainer. I don't believe in exercising for hours on end, nor do I even deprive myself. I actually do enjoy my desserts; my go-to indulgence is dark chocolate. But I do make a lot of intentional choices. And I follow a few very basic health tenets—and have done so for years.

The tenets I follow have helped me through a number of difficult moments in my life, such as my son Wyatt's brain cyst diagnosis and treatment. Indeed, we don't just need good health for all the good we want to accomplish. We need good health to give us the physical and emotional strength to absorb and respond gracefully to the least expected challenges.

That's what led me to write down my advice and start sharing it with others. That's how **Molly Vibrant Living** and the **21-Day Action Plan** came to be, followed by workshops and a host of private clients who wanted additional coaching.

21-DAY ACTION PLAN RESULTS

Thousands of people have now tried out the **Molly Vibrant Living** approach and embarked on the **21-Day Action Plan**. The results?

- On average, women lose three or four pounds a week, although many have lost more—11.5 to 18 pounds in three weeks. The average weight loss for men in 21 days is between 15 and 27 pounds.
- They often lose as many inches (in various measurements across their bodies) as pounds. Their clothes fit them more comfortably and they carry themselves differently.
- Nearly 99 percent of participants report feeling significantly more energetic within three or four days of starting the program.
- They *feel* better, experience fewer aches and pains, sleep better, and report better moods, greater confidence and comfort with their bodies. They feel sexier!
- On average, 98 percent of them plan more and create more intention in their lives. Writing daily in their 21-Day Daily Log helps keep them accountable and celebrates their short-term accomplishments, feeding their confidence in long-term achievement.

Haley, a 38-year-old mom and teacher, says that the **21-Day Action Plan** was "exactly what [she] needed to start exercising and eating better." She shares, "I am losing the big stomach I acquired over the last five years. I am so blessed to be alive and am feeling better than I ever have because of you."

Sue, a mother of four, lost 16-and-a-half pounds with the action plan. "I feel fantastic, energetic, accomplished and so on-track!" Sue relayed. "Getting my physical self in order has flowed into getting more disciplined in other areas of my life. *I'm not wasting calories and I'm not wasting time* . . . thank you, Molly."

Participants report better love lives, better sex and stronger relationships.

Here are 47-year-old Brandon's results: "I have more energy than I have had in years. Since doing your 21-Day program five months ago, I have lost 52 pounds and look like I did when I was 21. Seriously, everyone tells me that! I attribute my success to replacing soda with water, eating more vegetables and adding exercise to my life. Not only do I look better, but I feel great . . . Molly, you may even get the credit for me getting a girlfriend!"

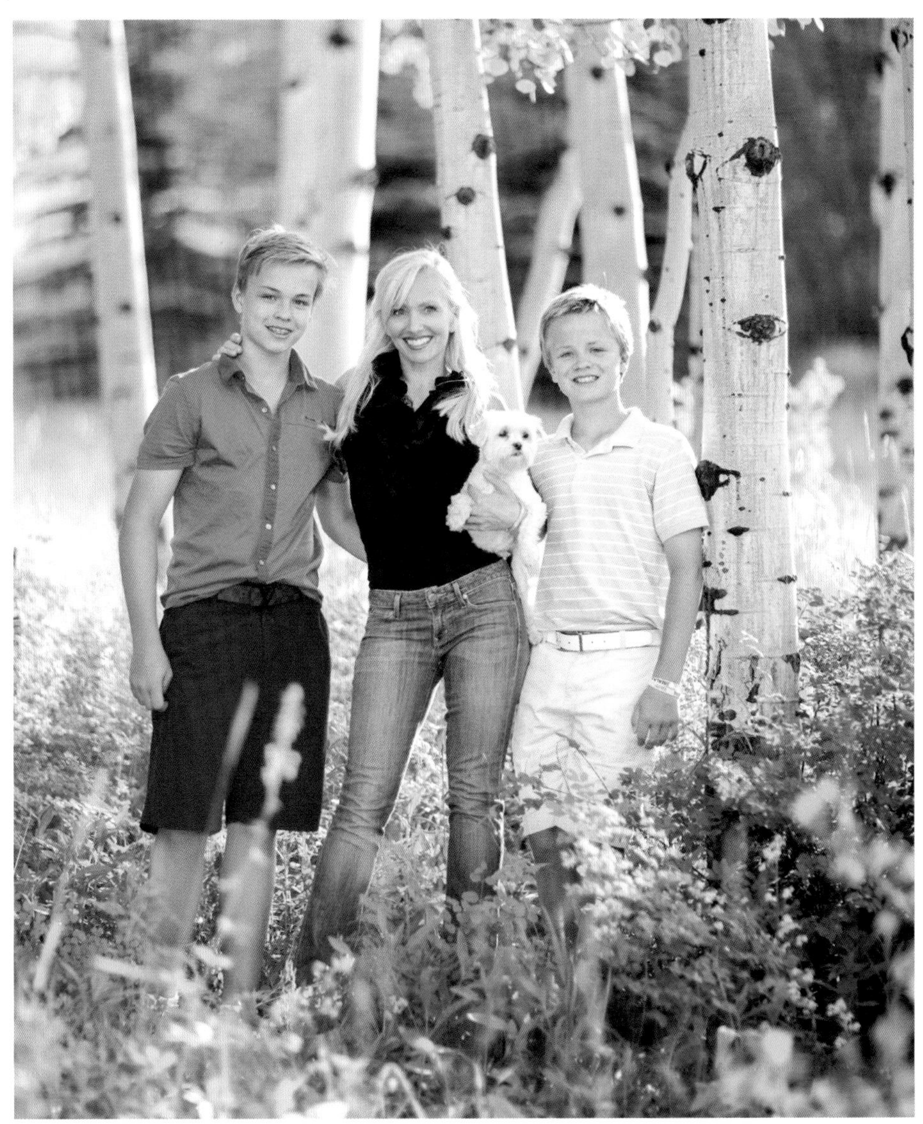

Among the aspen trees with my sons Spencer (left) and Wyatt (right)... and our dog Lizzie Mae.

Indeed, months after completing the **21-Day Action Plan**, clients and workshop participants write to tell me how much weight they have lost—and kept off—and how integral to their lives the plan's healthy habits have become. I also love hearing from clients about life goals they have already proudly achieved, not to mention how easily they can now name and imagine new goals for themselves.

WHY 21 DAYS?

Let's say, just for a moment, that you devoted three weeks of your life to retraining yourself. Twenty-one days is doable, right? It's an energy pilot experiment—a regimen in which you will drop weight, lose inches, feel better and start pursuing a life of more profound meaning and purpose.

Research suggests that it takes *about three weeks* to turn an act of self-control into a habit (that requires little or no thought). Someday, we hope neuroscientists will be able to tell us precisely how long it takes for tentative nerve-cell firing patterns to become "go-to synapses" that the brain readily calls upon. But 21 days seems to be the norm. After all, that's when the recipient of an artificial limb tells us a new appendage begins to feel natural, according to Dr. Maxwell Maltz, author of *Psycho-Cybernetics*.[1]

What's in store for you during this three-week plan? This isn't a strict and complicated diet, or a rigorous boot camp. Rather, **Molly Vibrant Living** relies on simple, practical tips to *invigorate* your body, *sharpen* your mind, *generate plentiful energy* and coax new and soulful ambitions into being. In this plan, you make simple replacements, substituting exercise, wholesome ingredients and selfless service for habits that are limiting you.

You can do this! Because the **21-Day Action Plan** is comprised of *only* four rules, or pillars, to follow. Your focus will be on hydration, moving your body, nutrient-rich eating and soul-expanding work. Together, these four pillars become super powers for your health, *right away* yielding surges in energy; within a couple of weeks, producing weight loss and mood stability; and within months and years, lending you enormous cancer-preventing and heart health-promoting benefits in addition to immeasurable joy and satisfaction.

HOW TO USE THE PLAN

Remember: This is *your* 21 days and it's up to you to decide what you want to accomplish during this period. This is not about achieving a fashion magazine's ideal of perfection. Most of us don't have the genetic makeup to be a size 4. And much of what we see from photo shoots is airbrushed anyway and has little to do with how real people look. That's why none of the photos in this book are Photoshopped. I'm a real person, and I want you to experience real health, tailored to your goals and your body.

Don't be tempted to delay the plan until a calmer period weeks or months from now. Each and every day, most of us will have difficulty reaching the goals we set for ourselves, with unique challenges and body types to overcome.

And life throws all of us curves. When I ask people in the workshops how many of them have experienced hardships or unexpected stresses in the last month, every hand in the room goes up, including mine. In the chapters to come, I will share the challenges I have faced—the ways that health problems and heartaches tried to knock me and my family for a loop.

Begin your **21-Day Action Plan** by reading pages 16-73. In these chapters, you'll find the Four Pillars that make up the **Molly Vibrant Living** program, 21-day success stories and more of my story, which I hope will serve as inspiration for your journey. *Commit to be Faithfully Fit* is my top 10 tips to help you devote yourself to a healthier lifestyle, and *Rules of Purposeful Engagement* will make a few details of the plan even clearer.

Planning is critical to your success. So the **21-Day Action Plan** section (pages 74–147) will help you set challenging but achievable goals for your health and well-being and put you in the frame of mind to achieve those goals. Review the *Prep List* (page 90) and take the recommended steps before you launch into keeping your *Daily Log* and tracking your progress.

One aspect that sets **Molly Vibrant Living** apart from other wellness efforts is the program's interactive nature. To begin your journey, I ask that you share your personal goals with me and activate your participation in the **21-Day Action Plan** by joining the **Vibrant Living Community** via my website: www.mollyshattuck.com. I will post daily messages, and you'll get to meet other members of the **Vibrant Living Community** who are also on the road to a healthier and fuller life. I urge you to interact with the participants, motivating and holding each other accountable as you integrate healthier practices into each day of your life.

LET'S GO!

It's time to get started! Work through the **21-Day Action Plan** *Daily Log* (pages 92–141), reading the comments and suggestions as well as recording your efforts. The focus of the **21-Day Action Plan** is to turn a few basic, but critically important actions into routines that will carry you forward. Writing down your progress each day is *the most important step* to forging healthy and sustainable habits.

The *Grocery List* and *Make REAL Meals* on pages 82 and 148 will be indispensable to you in stocking your kitchen with nutrient-rich ingredients and planning delicious, nourishing meals in the coming weeks and beyond.

You have made a decision to take control of your own health and create habits to support the quality of life you want to be living. Congratulations!

The author of the best-seller *Life's Little Instruction Book*, H. Jackson Brown, Jr., says "Opportunity dances with those already on the dance floor."

It's your turn to dance, letting good health restore your energy.

After three weeks, the plan is for you to be so invigorated that pinnacle moments appear to you as distinct possibilities. Go out and cultivate a life full of deliberate, purpose-driven choices. Reap all the energy you need to fulfill your dreams and bring your bright and brilliant light into the world.

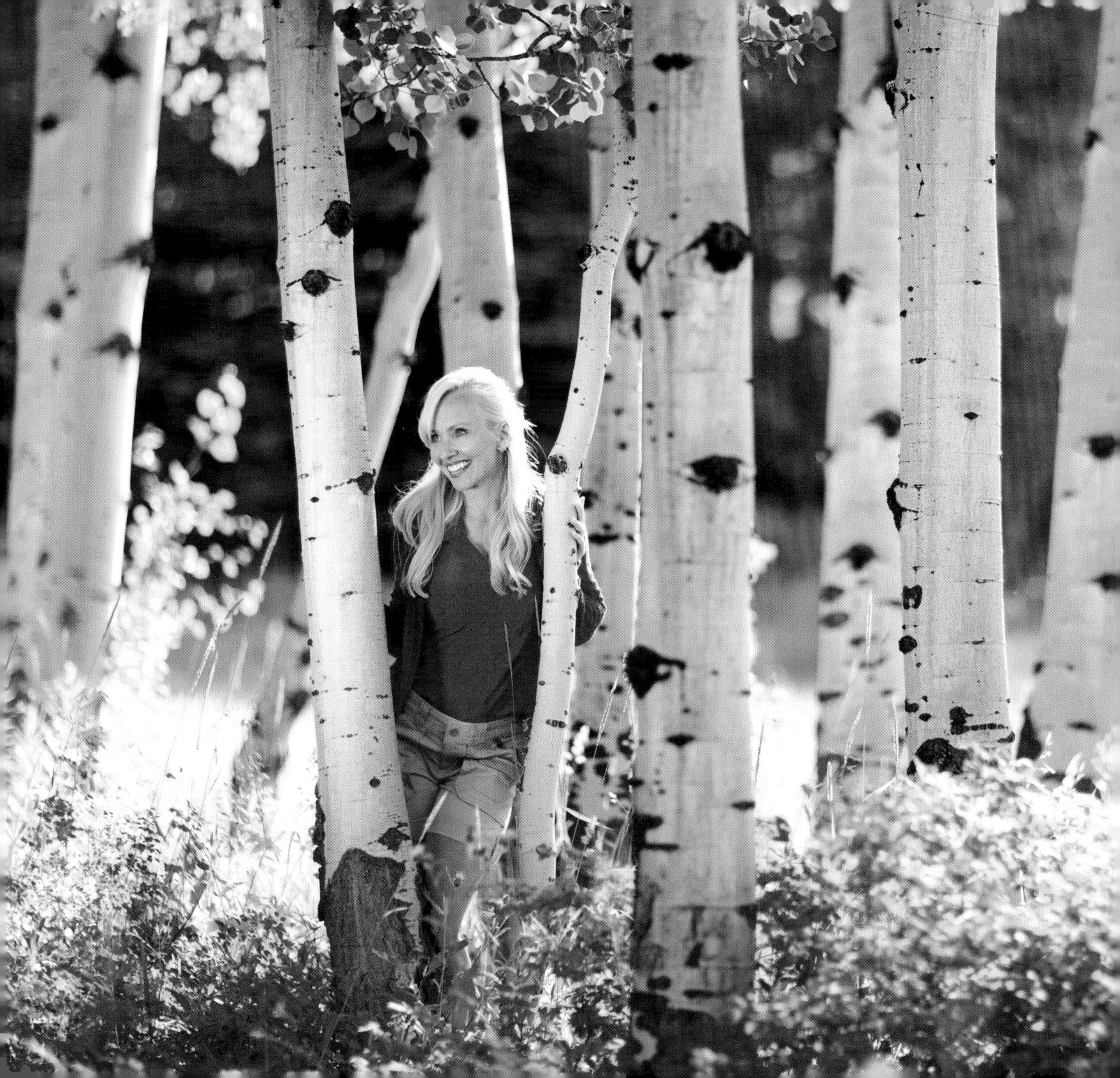

THE FOUR PILLARS

Learn the fundamentals and delve into the science behind living your life with better health and higher purpose.

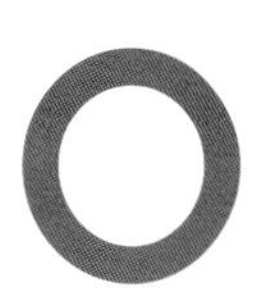

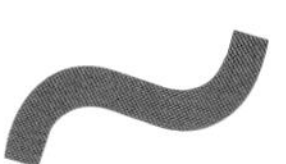

Drink Water

A MESSAGE OF SELF CARE & HIGH PURPOSE

"The rivers flow not past, but through us."
—*John Muir*

Indeed, water is at the very core of our existence.

Water covers about 70 percent of the earth's surface. We swim, bathe, exercise and play in it. We use it to grow our food, clean our homes, generate electricity and manufacture nearly everything we wear.

On average, an adult's body weight is made up of as much as 60 percent water.[2] Not surprisingly, water is an essential part of proper body functioning. It's the means for transporting nutrients to cells, hormones, and nervous impulses throughout the body. Water aids in digestion, circulation and body temperature regulation and it provides a moist environment for ear, nose and throat tissue. It elevates energy and can be critical to weight management. *Every system and vital organ in your body needs water for optimal performance.*

That's why drinking water is the first pillar in the Molly Vibrant Living program. It's also the one I tell clients never to skip.

WHY WATER WOWS ME

I grew up in a household in which we drank water and milk. For a special treat, the family would order pizza, which came with a 2-liter bottle of root beer. But not having it very often, I never got used to the carbonation. Drinking water, on the other hand, has always been an essential part of my life.

My "aha moment" about the power of water came in 1998 after the birth of my oldest child Spencer. I had gained 50 pounds during my pregnancy and was breastfeeding when I noticed that the more water I drank, the more milk I produced and the quicker the weight melted away. Seeing the body work so miraculously—giving birth to and feeding a child—this important lesson was impressed on me: *I am a vessel and I need to be filled first to effectively nurture life—my life, the life of my family and the living, breathing life force that God wants us—all of us—to be in the world.*

I truly believe that water transforms us. And that our bodies are vessels of living water, designed to convey goodness, strength and compassion. That's why my water bottle has become like an extra appendage. I take it to business meetings, to nice restaurants, even to church. At my Episcopalian church where we still get dressed up for services, my sports water bottle makes a bit of a statement in the pews.

It's possible I'm a wee bit fanatical about my water intake. In a restaurant, I've been known to ask for an empty glass into which I can pour the contents of my water bottle so I can keep tracking my water throughout the meal.

But before you discount the wacky water lady, understand this:

Of the four pillars, water is the most immediate game changer in the **21-Day Action Plan**. Literally, within two or three days of getting fully hydrated, people experience bursts of new energy.

WATER & OVERALL HEALTH

If you'll forgive the pun, the science of hydration is clear. Water is a marvelous multi-tasker in our bodies, organically contributing to our health in myriad ways.

Water is the big player in plasma, making up 90 percent of this fluid component of the blood. When you skimp on H_2O, the plasma gets thick, sluggish and less efficient, which, not surprisingly, is also the way you feel when you aren't properly hydrated.[3] If, alternatively, you like the sound of essential nutrients such as minerals, vitamins and glucose getting delivered to your cells quickly and reliably, water's just the carrier to do the job.

But water isn't done with you yet. It takes out your trash—literally—flushing toxins from your liver and other vital organs, and it breaks down the bio-chemicals of the food we eat. And water also regulates your temperature, something you need every day but is going to come in very handy during climate change.

A few years ago, workers at the Red Cross noticed that blood donors who drank 16 ounces of water before giving blood were a lot less likely to keel over and faint after they had given a pint. So the Red Cross went on to fund research at Vanderbilt University that showed that drinking water activates the sympathetic nervous system. Ahem, what else did the study show the multi-tasker does? It keeps us more alert, with slight blood pressure elevations, and it boosts energy.[4]

Depriving your body of water on a regular basis is, in essence, taking a Hercules of health and tying its hand behind its back. With inadequate hydration over long periods of time, you make your heart pump harder, elevating your blood pressure continually. With a prolonged water shortage, the body turns to the liver to do the jobs water used to do. And when the liver has to work overtime, more of the fat you consume gets stored rather than burned off.[5]

The brain is also about 80 percent water. As a result, even slight dehydration diminishes our ability to think clearly. Just imagine the consequences for our productivity and ingenuity if our workforce is chronically under-hydrated. Research shows that even mild to moderate levels of dehydration can impair our performance with tasks involving short-term memory, math, sensory and spatial perception, visual and psychomotor skills that we use to drive a car, throw a ball or any task that is largely physical.[6]

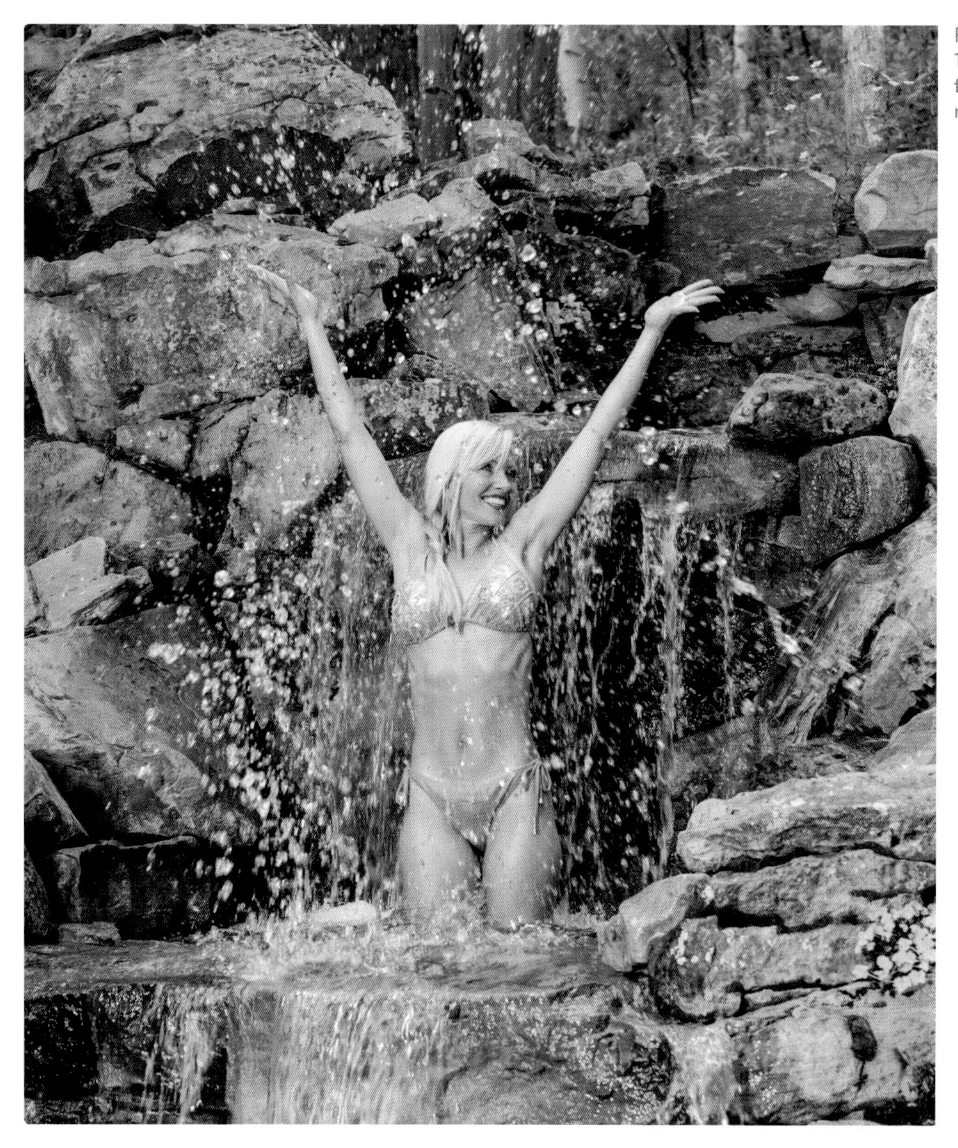

Replenish yourself! We lose 10 cups of water each day from our usual activities, even more with a rigorous workout.

So let's review. Dehydration can thicken and slow our blood. It holds trashy toxins in and hampers the breakdown of nutrients. It spikes our blood pressure and destabilizes our blood sugar. It leaves us hot, bothered, less coordinated and mentally fatigued. Sometimes dehydration brings on headaches and pangs of hunger shortly after we have eaten. It can also induce the desire to stretch out under your desk and snooze in the middle of a workday afternoon. If you're starting to resemble these remarks, drinking water is your best revenge.

HOW DOES WATER HELP WITH WEIGHT?

When you drink water, you also eat less. Yet I find that it is one of the least discussed strategies for losing weight. If you look at the major weight loss programs, you'll find water recommended deep within the instructions and not front and center, where thousands of Molly Vibrant Living water-guzzlers will tell you it belongs.

Dr. Mehmet Oz, the cardiothoracic surgeon so many of us tune into for sound medical advice, is emphatic about water's role in revving your metabolism. "When your body doesn't have enough water, your metabolism slows down," he says. "Drink water."[7]

It's proved life changing for Molly Vibrant Living clients to ask themselves, "Am I thirsty?" and "I want to eat, but is it possible I only need water?" After all, it's very common to mistake thirst for hunger.

That's why I always recommend 12 to 16 ounces of water at the start of a meal and particularly when you're thinking about having a snack *in between* meals. Not only does water help satisfy you, but the act of drinking causes you to contemplate the fat- or sugar-laden item you're about to put in your mouth. If you establish the habit of *always* drinking water before consuming food, you may rethink the urge to devour the *entire* brownie, you know, the one from the coffee cart that's bigger than your hand.

Adopting this habit can have a significant impact on your weight. Many studies have found that people who drink water before eating consume an average of 75 fewer calories per meal.[8]

Take that action twice a day and it could add up to a 14-pound weight loss in a single year.

HOW MUCH WATER, MOLLY?

Everyone's hydration threshold is different. For me, the sweet spot is 120 ounces—nearly twice the amount recommended by Weight Watchers, for example.[9] When I drink 120 ounces each day, I feel rested and energetic. If I get behind on my consumption, my system feels "off" and I tire quickly.

In my years of helping people get healthy, I have found that between 90 and 120 ounces has a dramatic impact on the way people look and feel. Nearly all of the women and men who have completed the 21-Day Action Plan and followed my recommendations for water consumption tell me they have more energy, are less hungry, see an improvement in the appearance of their skin, and simply feel better overall. It's hard to argue with results like that.

We've all heard the advice to drink eight 8-ounce glasses of water a day for good health. The "8 by 8" rule remains popular because it's easy to remember. But the Institute of Medicine guidelines on total water intake are more specific.

FILL UP WITH FACTS

You are the vessel! Establish your routine of healthy hydration with these practical pointers:

- Start drinking water the moment you wake up in the morning and throughout the day. If you feel thirsty, chances are you're already dehydrated, so you may want to increase the rate at which you are drinking. Try 30 ounces before breakfast, 30 ounces after breakfast and before lunch, and another 30 ounces after lunch and before dinner. Consume more after dinner but be sure to stop drinking at least an hour prior to bedtime.
- Drink 12-16 ounces of water before every meal and snack, and even more if you're still hungry after eating.
- Keep a 30-ounce water bottle with you at all times. Make it *impossible* to have an excuse not to drink water. Go to www.mollyshattuck.com for all your hydration products.
- Fill up your bottle when it's empty, not half full, to more accurately track your consumption.
- If you neglect to consume 90 ounces or more of water during the day and you're heading out to dinner, take your bottle with you and pour the contents in the restaurant's glass to track your intake.
- If you're having an alcoholic beverage, follow it up with a glass of water. (Alcohol and caffeine are diuretics, which can lead to dehydration.) Limit yourself to one glass of alcohol per week while trying to get healthier, and always alternate an alcoholic beverage with a glass of water.
- Drink water before, during, and after exercise to replenish what you've lost through perspiration. With increased hydration comes increased energy!
- For a jolt of flavor, garnish your water with a slice of lemon, lime, orange, cucumber, watermelon or a few berries.
- Over-consumption of water is a rare occurrence for adults who eat a healthy diet, according to research at the Mayo Clinic. However, it's unnecessary to gulp 100 ounces at once. Get in the habit of drinking filtered or safe-drinking tap water throughout the day.
- Drinking water leads to glowing skin and a better complexion. When you're well hydrated, your skin cells plump up due to improved circulation. The same holds true for cardiovascular exercise—that's why we get the flush cheeks. Even Dr. Margaret E. Parsons, a spokeswoman for the American Academy of Dermatology, acknowledges that when skin is dehydrated, "fine wrinkles certainly seem to show up a bit more."
- Finally, three cups of coffee in the morning or two glasses of iced tea does not equate to proper hydration. *Just drink plain, filtered water.*

Dr. Leigh Vinocur, a board certified emergency room physician at the University of Maryland School of Medicine, encourages us to rely on the Institute's recommendations that women drink 60 ounces of water each day, or "a total of 91 ounces (that's about 2.7 liters) per day—from all food and beverages combined. For men, it's about 125 ounces a day (or 3.7 liters) from all sources." If you are an older adult, or taking medication that affects your thirst mechanism, such as medicines for heart conditions, stomach ulcers or depression, you may need to fill your glass even more often.[10] And finally, I also have heard numerous doctors recommend that a person should drink half their body weight in ounces of water.

So how can you gauge if you're getting enough water to bolster your body, brain and metabolism? Dr. Vinocur says your urine will be fairly clear, not a darker shade of yellow.

A NATION OF CHRONIC DEHYDRATION

If you have a thirsty feeling, you are already dehydrated. Once again, this question—*Am I thirsty?*—triggers a realization many of my clients say they rarely considered before joining the Molly Vibrant Living program.

Truly, we are a nation of chronic dehydration, with roughly 75 to 80 percent of Americans going day after day with too little fluid in their bodies. According to the Centers for Disease Control and Prevention, 43 percent of adults drink fewer than four cups of water a day, including 7 percent who drink no water at all on any given day.[11]

It's true, water bottles are now ubiquitous, much more a part of our everyday lives than they used to be. But if you are downing two 12-ounce bottles of water each day, you are replenishing less than a third of the amount you lose each day through normal body functions such as breathing, sweating and going to the bathroom. You literally lose 10 cups of day, and that's without working out!

Before we go further, I know all this talk about hydration is making some of you want a Big Gulp™ soda or a Venti™ mocha with whip. (See "Fill Up with Facts" for the low-down on substitutes.) But stay with me for now, so you can hear from a client for whom water has proved life-changing.

MARTA'S STORY

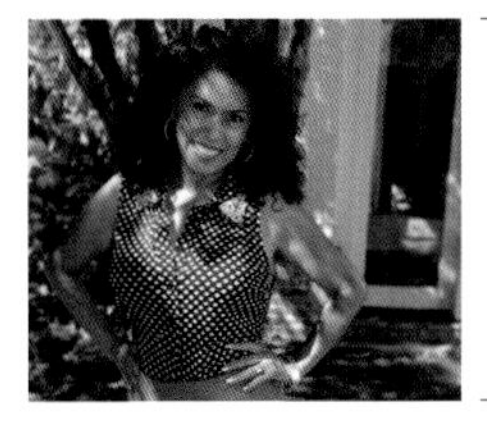

Marta
AGE 56
OCCUPATION Assistant, Child Caregiver, Preschool Teacher, and Hairstylist
HOMETOWN Laurel, MD

Two and a half years ago, Marta joined one of the 21-Day Challenges (what they used to be called) in Baltimore. At that time, she experienced a great deal of fatigue, struggling many mornings to get out of bed. Often Marta left her exercise class at her gym before it was finished, and she would just stop in the middle of bike rides with her husband. She didn't have energy to do things she loved and had gained weight over the years.

Yet almost as soon as the 56-year-old wife, mother, preschool teacher and hairstylist learned about the pillar of drinking water, she became a devotee. "I saw the results." Within two days, before the other four pillars had time to take hold, Marta said, "My energy was higher."

Marta lost 12 pounds within the 21-day span. She continued to lose weight afterwards, "without even thinking about it," because by then, the four pillars were ingrained in her. But the way she *feels* is even more compelling. No more dragging herself out of bed. "Today, I'm up before it's time to get up. Physically, my energy level is much higher. I feel like I did in my 20's."

Marta says, "I remember Molly emphasizing—preaching, as I like to call it—that if we did nothing else to improve our health, we had to drink a lot of water." So now, when people ask Marta how she has the energy to bike 35 miles with her husband or start and finish the craft projects she enjoys, she says, "If you do nothing else, drink a lot of water. I preach to them, too."

Furthermore, Marta says, "I haven't had a cold in two years." When she starts to feel a sore throat coming on, Marta starts increasing her water. "Water just seems to be my medicine."

FILL YOURSELF UP

Go ahead, fill yourself with sips of water throughout the day. See where your sweet spot is, on the spectrum between 90 and 120 ounces over the course of the day.

How does this habit sound to you now, this idea of pausing, pausing again, pausing frequently throughout the day to take sips and gulps of water?

And refill your water bottle with clean, filtered water. (For more practical tips, see "Fill Up with Facts" on page 20.) Can you conceive of taking care of yourself every day in this attentive way?

My experience has been that many clients, women in particular, feel selfish about taking time to take care of themselves. Sometimes our lives are so full, attending to the needs of others, that we resist even taking bathroom breaks. And you are going to need a few more bathroom breaks if you are filling up with 90 ounces of toxin-flushing, organ-cleansing water every day.

GIVE YOURSELF PERMISSION

In this way, I've learned that this simple edict to drink water can be very "loaded." I think that's because water represents a really basic form of self-care that many of us—in this nation of chronic dehydration—do not afford ourselves.

When stresses complicate our lives—perhaps job demands or the responsibility of caring for aging parents, difficulties in a marriage or economic strains—we often respond with work and worry that becomes consuming. We sleep less, and fatigue—combined with stress—often prompts us to binge eat. We exercise less and we pound coffee and energy drinks to recoup flagging energy. Sometimes we go on this way for weeks and months on end, triggering devastating effects on our bodies, our weight, and our moods.

Strangely, in these times, we don't give ourselves permission to attend to the lifeblood of energy and health we most need to draw upon. I wish I could write everyone a note to take to the principal. Or a note to

BUT WHAT ABOUT OTHER DRINKS!?

Hands down, water is the best choice when you're thirsty. It's both calorie- and chemical-free, and choosing water over other beverages can significantly reduce your calorie intake while detoxifying your body. It's also cheap! Try saving the money you would spend on sodas and $5 fancy coffee drinks. You may end up being able to afford a vacation or, at least, a fabulous pair of shoes!

Worried you will miss out on vitamin C you usually consume in juice? Choose water and a fresh orange or handful of strawberries. Juice is high in concentrated sugar while lacking the fiber that's critical for keeping your system running smoothly.

Looking for a thirst-quencher during and after a hard workout? Choose water, not sports or energy drinks, many of which contain excess caffeine, sugar, and other chemicals.

Replacing calorie-loaded sugary drinks with water can have a huge impact on your weight. But the same holds true for diet drinks. New research is revealing that artificial sweeteners in diet sodas and other calorie-free, flavored beverages can actually raise your insulin levels and lower your blood sugar. This, in turn, stimulates hunger and moves existing calories into your fat cells.[12]

Replacing diet or carbonated, artificially flavored beverages and alcohol with water can help you lose up to 20 pounds in a single year, even if you make no other changes to your eating habits.[13] If you *really* enjoy sodas and alcohol, take a disciplined approach and limit yourself to one cup a day, period. By limiting your intake, you'll lose weight and clear your body of harmful chemicals.

Also, keep in mind that alcohol often goes hand in hand with unhealthy eating, as we tend to lose self-control after a few cocktails. Keep your alcohol consumption in check, and you'll stay in charge of *everything* you put into your mouth.

Finally, not all drinking water is created equal. Drink filtered water and if you have to drink bottled, be sure to do due-diligence on which ones are actually filtered.

The most important thing to remember is that adequate hydration is a healthy habit, one that requires *intentional* action to establish. Make a BPA-free water bottle your constant companion, and start keeping track of your intake during your **21-Day Action Plan** and beyond.

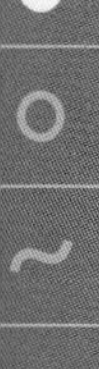

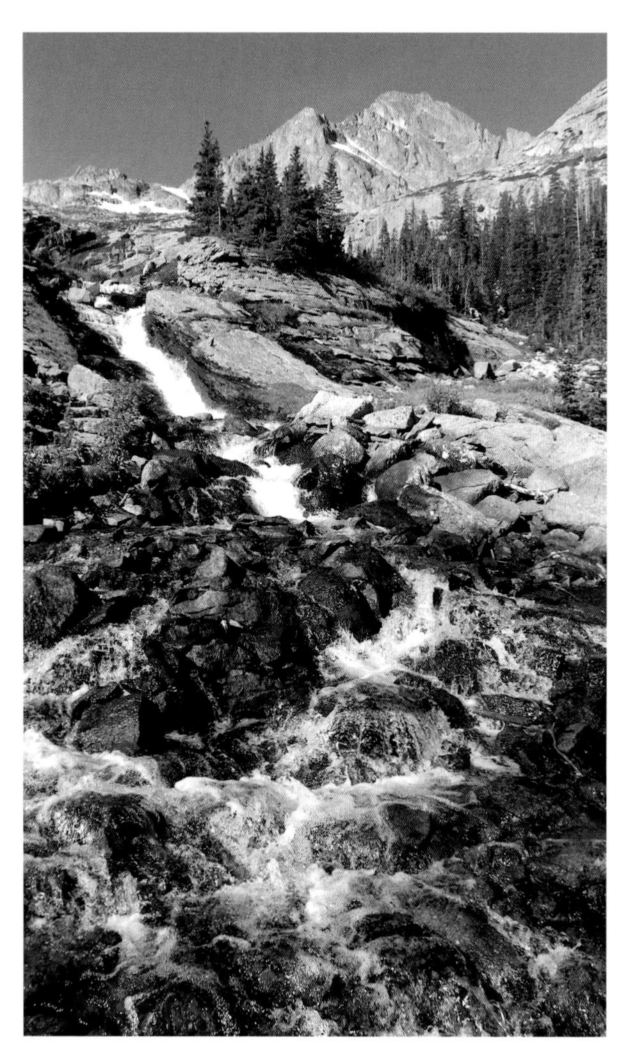

My sister, Lisa, took this stunning photo in Colorado during one of our hikes.

that stubborn naysayer in your mind who says you don't deserve to take time to care for yourself. *Listen, naysayer:* Your health is the most valuable asset in your possession. You need to invest in its well-being. You are a child of God and you richly deserve to slow down a little every day and fill yourself.

Strive to drink 90 ounces each day. Water *cleanses* your body by flushing your system; it refreshes you as it's the only liquid that truly quenches your thirst; it *satisfies* you throughout the day so you don't overeat; and it naturally *energizes* you by keeping you alert and well hydrated. If you do *nothing* else to get yourself healthier, drink your water.

Pause. Think. Act. This prescription for health and life will appear again and again in this book.

As a pillar, "drink water" sounds like a fairly innocuous edict. But when you incorporate the steps to higher hydration—pause, think and act—you begin to chip away at a swarm of behaviors associated with unhealthy and mindless living.

In my experience, being hydrated keeps me alert and calm, better able to attend to problems that come up and to respond gracefully. And filling yourself in the ways this program will ask you to—first with water and then with other nutrients and behaviors—is not selfish. It's actually *selfless and sacred*.

HONOR YOUR BODY, HONOR GOD

Honoring your body is a very faithful way of responding to your creator. Those of us who were baptized—as infants, children or adults—were marked with water, a cross fingered on our foreheads or our bodies immersed in a pool. Baptism is a blessing of our bodies, a ritual of God's protection and caretaking of us. With water, we are initiated into a lifelong search for the sacred purpose of our lives.

Every day you live, you have a chance to fill your vessel in a fundamentally healing way—to thank God for water, the source of all life. And to renew your baptism, a vow to keep your body strong and holy, and to keep seeking the higher purpose of life that God intends for you.

A few years ago, my family and I were on a boat in Casco Bay when a sudden squall came up. The boat was full of children and adults, my kids among those in the front of the boat, all in life preservers. Out of nowhere, the waves came at us hard. And several times the boat crested and fell with a violent smack against the surge.

In one of these cycles, my seven-year-old daughter Lillian was thrown up in the air and then fell, hitting the boat with great force as it came up from its plunge. I witnessed all of this from my seat behind her, Lillian's face immediately wrenching in pain. She had broken her back, I seemed to realize almost instantly.

Lillian was struggling to breathe, and a rescue in these conditions was not going to happen quickly. But instinctively, I seemed to understand that Lillian needed to be kept still and straight. Since there was nowhere safe to get her prone, I stretched myself out like a plank for her to lie on. That way, I could absorb the force of the waves, and promote a stillness that enabled her to breathe.

Within an hour, a Coast Guard cutter made its way to us and medics came aboard to transport Lillian to the hospital. They used my body, still and straight, as the stretcher to lift Lillian out of the boat. She has since made a full recovery from the spinal break.

We never know in life when we will be called on to be the conduit for higher purpose, when we will need a reserve of clear thinking or of physical strength to survive a squall.

With these four pillars, I do pray that you will see your body as the splendid gift that it is, a vessel you are disciplined about replenishing and from which you can pour your love into the world.

Eat REAL

A MESSAGE OF CONNECTION & GRATITUDE

"Humankind has not woven the web of life. We are but one thread within it. Whatever we do to the web, we do to ourselves. All things are bound together. All things connect."
—*Chief Seattle*

It was a Friday evening and my children and I were serving dinner at Baltimore Station, a residential treatment program for military veterans and others trying to move out of poverty, addiction and homelessness. The kids were lined up behind the buffet. My oldest, Spencer, served the chicken, the middle child, Wyatt, the bread and my youngest, Lillian, the green beans. One by one, the men came through the line and we filled their plates with colorful, savory vegetables and protein we had prepared just for them.

One man stopped Lillian before she could scoop the beans onto his plate. "What is that?" he asked. "They're green beans," Lillian replied, "Would you like some?" Tentatively, the man accepted on his plate only a couple of the long and vividly green beans.

Another man came though the line and, again, just at Lillian's station, stopped to ask, "What is that?" And before we finished, Lillian got the question several more times, which she found very puzzling. What was it about her dish that provoked so many questions? One of the men gestured, showing Lillian the small size of the green beans he was used to seeing. Another gentleman said the beans looked almost neon, nothing like the ones he'd eaten before.

I explained to Lillian that the men were accustomed to a canned, precut type. Despite being middle aged or older, few of them had experienced the color, the length, or the snap of a farm fresh green bean. Yet, these same men, the ones who had raised an eyebrow at this odd looking veggie, returned for seconds and thirds of Lillian's beautiful beans.

REAL FOOD IS JOY ON A PLATE

For me, there is profound joy in preparing, eating and sharing REAL food. Sitting down with the men at the shelter that night, my kids and I experienced how *alive* fresh and wholesome food can be and how for some, it's a rare *gift*. We brought the best that the earth had to offer and it nourished the men, and all of us, body and soul.

If you have a garden from which you pluck herbs or vegetables, or if you've shopped at a local farmers' market, you may have experienced this, too. When it is newly picked, a carrot or a berry bursts with a kind of lively, earthy vibration—almost like a pulse. And the lucky people who get to taste the food that still carries those vibrations are enlivened by them, too.

That's why the second pillar is REAL food, building on the foundation of hydration.

WHAT IS REAL FOOD?

Real food is from the earth, or very lightly processed. It is not filled with preservatives and chemicals—the names of which we'd be hard pressed to read, recognize or pronounce. Eating REAL, as I urge you to do in the 21-Day Action Plan, means bending earthward and getting back to basics.

Focus on whole foods (fresh vegetables and fruit, whole grains, beans, legumes, lean meats, nuts, seeds and fish) and limit processed foods—those that come in a box, can, bag or jar with a barcode.

Wake up each day, determined to fill your body with as much color as nature—not Madison Avenue and major manufacturers—affords us. Take in the deep evergreen of kale and spinach; the royal purple of beets and plums; the poppy red of the red pepper and the flirty pinky-red of a raspberry.

Ask yourself these questions each day:

- Am I eating items rich in nutrients, or am I ingesting empty calories?
- Am I picking the God-given and earth-grown, or am I reaching for man-made convenience foods?
- Am I fueling my energy and higher purpose, or am I sapping it?

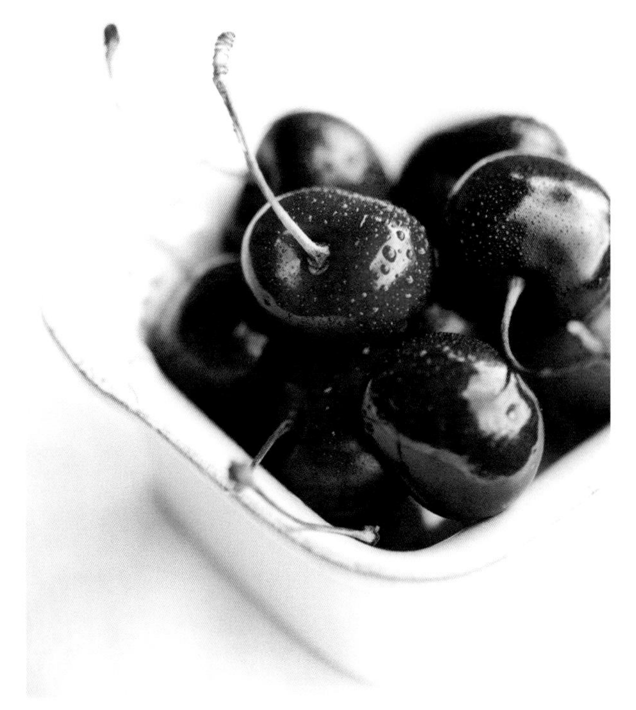

Start your day with breakfast—and include fruit to get a jump on your five daily servings of fruits and veggies.

HEALTHY POINTERS FOR A LIFE OF HEALTHY EATING

Below are additional considerations to ensure you're controlling overall food consumption and getting the nutrition you need for vitality and good health:

- Pasta tastes great, but it has little nutritional value unless you are consuming whole grain or high fiber varieties. Barilla Plus™ is my favorite. Satisfy your craving by allowing yourself 1 cup of this healthier option occasionally, served on a bed of fresh spinach and topped with steamed vegetables. You can also substitute quinoa or spaghetti squash for pasta. See *Make REAL Meals* (page 148) for ideas.
- Eat salad with veggies frequently *but* choose olive oil vinaigrette for dressing. Always have it in a separate dish on the side, whether at home or when dining out. Dip your fork into the dressing and then into your salad instead of pouring it on top. You'll eat less of the dressing this way.
- Cut your food before you eat. Doing so fools your mind into thinking you have more of the food than you do. Try it with an apple, a sandwich or even a cookie. You will get fuller more quickly, as I know and as researchers now tell us.[14]
- Minimize your intake of sodium- and fat-laden junk food like potato chips. Once you start eating, it's hard to stop. But if you do choose to indulge, never eat out of the bag. Instead, place one serving (as indicated on package) in a small dish. After eating, drink 12 gulps of water then brush your teeth. Do not return to the temptation.
- Avoid fried foods. Allow yourself one exception like French fries once a week if they are something you absolutely love and crave. Eat fresh-cut fries with the nutritious skin on and limit yourself to a serving size of seven. See *Make REAL Meals* (page 148) for a quick, easy and yummy recipe.
- Incorporate avocados, olive oil, almonds and walnuts into your diet several times a week.
- Avoid fatty cuts of red meat and processed meats with preservatives. They are loaded with unhealthy fat and linked to increased risks of cancer and diabetes. If you do occasionally indulge, grass-fed beef is considerably leaner than conventionally raised.
- Choose whole-grain breads over white bread and brown rice or quinoa over white rice.
- Eat vegetables raw, steamed or roasted with a drizzle of olive or avocado oil for flavor. Avoid boiling them—most of the nutrients will be poured down the sink. Your body actually absorbs more iron and other nutrients from dark, leafy greens like broccoli, green beans and spinach if you lightly steam them or sauté them in a small amount of oil.[15]
- Limit the amount of sugar you consume. It can be as addictive as some serious drugs, has little nutritional value, can be damaging to your teeth, and is loaded with calories.
- Increase the amount of fiber you eat because it aids in digestion and provides a feeling of fullness.

Really, the way we feed our bodies has a profound impact on who we are, how we feel and look, and our ability to lead fulfilling lives.

Delicious food is one of life's great pleasures, but it also has a very important job to do. It fuels our bodies with the ingredients we need for energy and good health. The daily choices you make about food are *medicinal in nature*. If you think about it, *you choose* three or four times a day whether you want to feel good or more lethargic. Whether you want to lose weight or gain weight. Whether you want to combat your risk of health problems such as high cholesterol or diabetes, or heighten the risks. Brighten your mood or darken it. Get your mojo back or kiss it goodbye. So *pause, think and act* with all these choices in mind.

Eating real requires us to be *keenly aware* of connections—of the connection between what we eat and how we feel, of the connection between each bite we take and the body we are powering, and of the connection between the farmer, the field and the food on our plates.

AUTOPILOT & ASLEEP AT THE WHEEL

Sadly, modern day eating often feels wildly disconnected from these truths. Eating has become an excessive indulgence for many people, with 68 percent of Americans overweight or obese.[16] I wish I could sugar coat it for you, but sugar coating is the reason many of us crave this junk in the first place.

When it comes to overeating and poor eating choices, it is as if our country is asleep at the wheel. We are careening out of control, fueling destructive behaviors. Too often, we allow gluttony and emotional eating, rather than true hunger, to dictate what we put in our mouths. The results? Weight gain, fatigue and a cycle that perpetuates a less active life.

OK, about now, you are probably thinking: How can we bump this cheerleader off her giant soapbox and let us eat our Cheetos™ in peace? But it's about to *get real*, with scientists weighing in on our eating habits and their devastating effects on the health of the world.

LET'S LOOK AT THE NUMBERS

A decade ago, the World Health Organization identified processed foods as the culprit in an international surge of obesity and chronic disease.[17] Internationally, more than 1.4 billion of us are overweight, and 300 million of us obese, according to the WHO website.[18] Clearly, this warning about fake food needs a much bigger siren.

Nearly 70 percent of the American diet is made up of processed food: crackers, cookies, chips, cereals, breakfast bars, soda and all the other stuff in the center aisles of the grocery store, be it Wal-Mart or Whole Foods. Processed food burns into our wallets, too, as it eats up 90 percent of our grocery spending in the United States.[19] From the industry's standpoint, this amounts to $850 billion each year.[20]

In the United States, we have been processing food for roughly 100 years, mostly to promote safety, shelf-life and appeal. But in the last 50 years, the processing has become extreme.[21] Indeed, there are now thousands of chemicals added to food products, many of which are untested. The health consequences are proving profound:

Diabetes: As a result of extreme processing, many foods contain advanced glycation endproducts, or

AGEs. Research has suggested that AGEs promote oxidative stress and inflammation within the body, which may in turn cause insulin resistance and lead to type 2 diabetes.[22]

In one study conducted by the Mount Sinai School of Medicine, two groups of mice were fed the same amount of calories. One group's diet contained AGEs while the other's did not. The study found that the mice who took in AGEs not only had lower antioxidant levels, higher body fat and more inflammation when compared to the other group, but they also exhibited premature insulin resistance, which suggests that AGEs may play a part in the development of diabetes.

Heart Disease: Many processed foods contain big no-no's for your heart and vascular health. Trans fats are very dangerous to our tickers but remain pervasive in common foods like margarine and spreads, cake and pancake mixes, canned soups, fast food and frozen entrées. Processed products are also loaded with sodium, hurting your heart and exposing you to an increased risk of stroke.

Cancer: A diet that's big on processed meats like hot dogs and sausages raises your cancer risk, as does a heavy reliance on refined carbohydrates like white flour, sugar and high fructose corn syrup. Same goes for vegetable oils, soft drinks and foods that are highly heated in oil such as French fries and potato chips, staples of the American diet.

As much as we enjoy the convenience of food that comes out of boxes or crinkly bags, the long-term effects—having to cope with earlier onset diabetes, heart disease and cancer—are anything but convenient.

To me, all this boils down to one thing: we need to get real about what we eat. We need more humility and less hubris when it comes to food and its role in our lives. We need to get back to thinking of food as something sacred, alive and transforming.

GRACE & GRATITUDE

You see, my other quirk, other than carrying my water bottle everywhere, is saying grace whenever I eat, even if it is just a snack. I say grace in public, in the presence of total strangers, and I say it in the privacy of my home with my family. There really isn't anywhere off limits for a prayer of thanksgiving, and that's what real food invokes in me—a sense that I am very, very fortunate and that God has provided life-sustaining food to me in the form of green leafy vegetables, delicious buttery salmon and tangy citrus. At its best, food is love—made manifest.

Even the creation story makes this clear. The Hebrew translation of the Garden of Eden account abounds with beautiful puns:

- The guy we know as Adam derives from the Hebrew "adamah" or earth and dust from the ground. Adamah also means arable land or fertile soil. We are, the Bible tells us, made from farmland!
- The word for "till" also means to serve. Charged with tilling the garden, the nature of our work is to not to push dirt around. It's to help, to shore up and to respond—in love.
- Eden, of course, means delight. Because there is tremendous joy to be found in the work of tilling, serving and appreciating the garden.

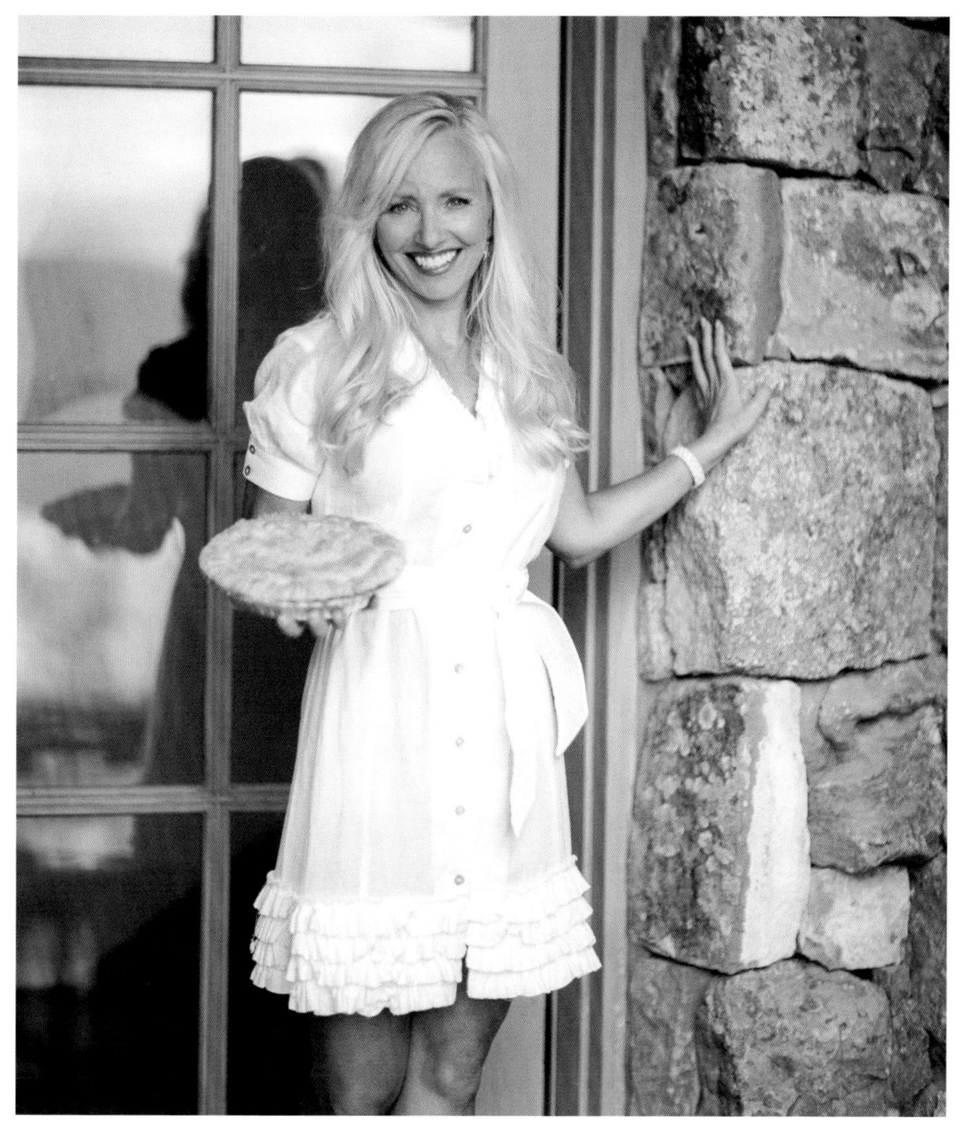

Cultivate a life in which you cook and bake for family, friends and neighbors. Reduce your reliance on prepackaged and processed cuisine.

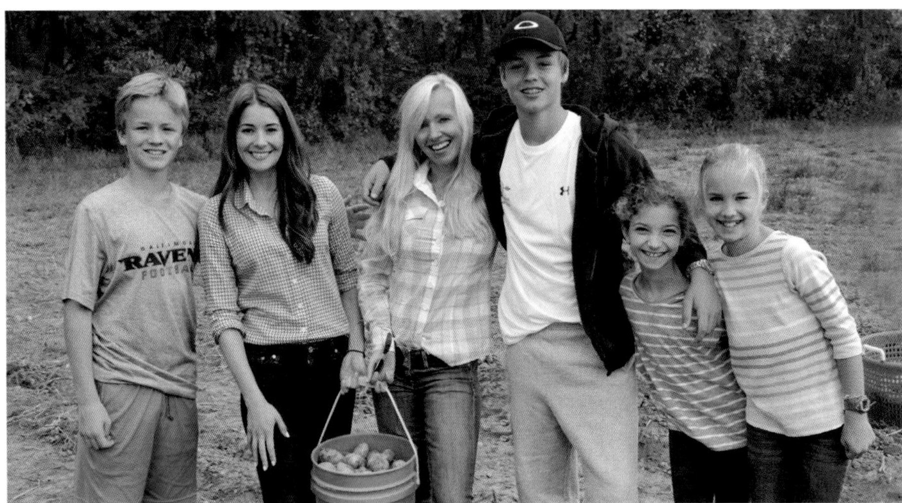

Harvesting vegetables at First Fruits Farm with my children, one of their friends, and nutritionist Katy Stephens. With 70 other volunteers, we harvested more than 50,000 pounds of food this day and donated it all to people in need of fresh food.

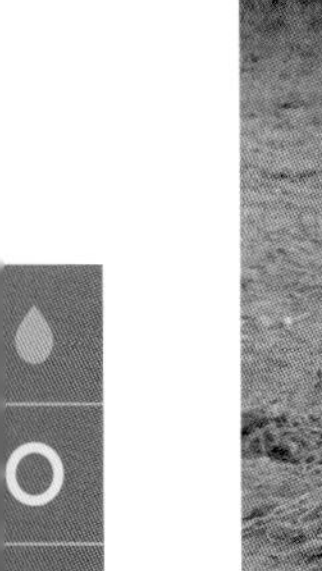

Being grateful for your food and saying so, whether you credit God or the earth for these blessings, is life-changing. It aligns your eating with a higher purpose—that of serving your body, of delighting in nourishing others and of expressing the deep connection we have to the earth of which we are all made.

When we experience ourselves as stewards of a splendid earth, a universe far bigger and more majestic than we are, it changes everything. You live a real life, without resorting to the excesses touted in our society.

A REAL WORLD APPROACH

With the first pillar, I asked you to learn to be generous with self-care, filling your vessel everyday with water. But with the second pillar, that of real food, I'm encouraging you to plant yourself firmly on God's green earth and *avoid extremism*.

In the 21-Day Action Plan, I am *not* asking you to become a vegetarian or live by kale smoothies alone. You don't have to go all Paleo or Atkins. You don't have to live without gluten, unless of course you have celiac disease or another medical condition that merits it. In the 21-Day Action Plan, you will enjoy stocking your fridge and trying recipes that are simple, clean and colorful (See the *Grocery List* on page 82 and the *Make REAL Meals* on page 148.)

By eating real, you avoid faddish and extreme approaches to dieting, from high-protein to low-carb or no-carb. These radical eating trends come and go, but in the process, they complicate your life unnecessarily and ultimately do more harm than good to your overall health.

It's dizzying sometimes, trying to discern how best to eat—which foods, when to eat and in what combination. The information can be confusing and misleading! However, understanding the essential foods needed for survival, we can remove the mystery around what to eat without sacrificing certain key nutrients.

THE SKINNY ON EATING FOR HEALTH & ENERGY

Let's break it down. The three main sources of nutrients come from *lean proteins, carbohydrates and fats*. According to the American Heart Association, these nutrients are the main dietary building blocks for healthy growth and development, including metabolism regulation.

Lean protein helps build and repair muscles, particularly during and after exercise. When you eat lean proteins such as chicken, fish, lean cuts of red meat, beans and low-fat dairy, you stay fuller and satisfied longer—wahoo! This fullness, in turn, decreases the amount of fat you consume and helps regulate your blood sugar levels. (Fewer afternoon headaches, less afternoon fatigue!)

You need carbohydrates such as fruits and vegetables, as well as complex carbohydrates such as whole grains, beans and legumes, so that you have fuel to burn throughout the day—to propel you through that interminably long meeting with an interminably long-winded peer, or through the really long line at the shoe sale, whichever you prefer. Carbohydrates also give us the energy we need for exercise, sex and everything else we need to get physical to do.

In moderation you do need some unsaturated (healthy) fat every day, including olive oil, avocados, nuts, chia and flax seeds. "Fat" is often blamed for health problems, including weight gain. But for mood, energy and mental clarity, for cardiovascular health and good cholesterol as well as for the absorption of vitamins A, D, E and K, unsaturated fat is our friend. The American Heart Association provides good guidelines on how much to eat.

On the other hand, fat-free and low-fat packaged foods *are not* your friends. These products are loaded with sodium, fat, sugar, and chemicals. Scientists are still studying their effects, but it appears that artificial sweeteners may inspire more sugar cravings, the very thing you wanted to avoid!

Should you buy organic? Experts recommend spending most of your organic food dollars (when possible and the budget allows) on produce and foods you eat most often. Locally grown food is also another route when sourcing and shopping because these foods tend to be fresher and kinder to the environment versus foods that have been picked too early, forced to ripen with chemicals and gases and transported across the country. Organic meats and dairy are hormone- and antibiotic-free, a fact you should consider to avoid unnecessary contamination to your body.

Eating real is not just about *what* you eat, it's also about *how* you eat. If you're concerned about your weight, don't make the common mistake of skipping meals to cut calories. This slows your metabolism and backfires in the long term. You'll eventually become ravenous and end up bingeing on foods that are full of fat and sodium. I strongly encourage you to plan your day so you can eat at least every three to four hours. (For more, see your *Plan to Eat Real* on pages 39-40.)

Consistent, quality nourishment will lend you consistent, quality energy and you'll rapid-burn calories, too, with a better metabolism.

CAN YOU REALLY DO IT?

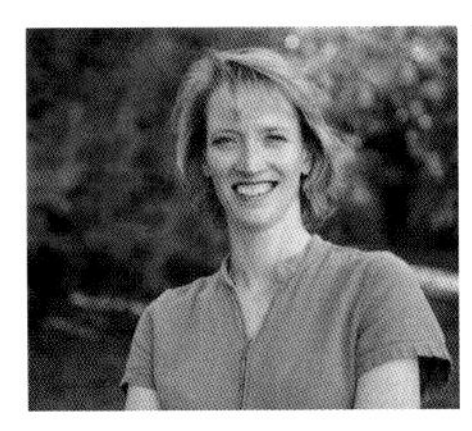

Leslie
AGE 40
OCCUPATION Executive Assistant
HOMETOWN Catonsville, MD

What would it take for you to incorporate these eating habits in your life? How does it sound to you, this idea of preparing food "from scratch" rather than relying on pre-mixed boxes and bags for dinner? Can you conceive of eating out less so that you can better control the amount of processed food you eat? Could you make room in your schedule for a bit more planning and shopping for fresh ingredients?

Tall and slim, Leslie Tinker appeared to be the picture of health when she joined a Molly Vibrant Living workshop in January 2013. But at 40, she was already experiencing the uncomfortable consequences of a poor diet, and had consulted five different gastroenterologists in her quest for better health.

A colonoscopy had revealed diverticulosis, in which pouches form in the colon that are magnets for infection; gastritis, an inflammation of her stomach; hemorrhoids, acid reflux and other effects of chronic constipation. Tears in her rectum made it painful to go to the bathroom and she was itchy and uncomfortable every day. What treatment had been recommended? Her doctor said, "All of these conditions are related to your diet."

Leslie, an executive assistant for a university philanthropy program, says, "I used to cook but it wasn't *real cooking*. I was shopping and eating from the 'middle of the store.' Everything was prepackaged—Hamburger Helper®, Shake N Bake® pork chops and sloppy joes." For side dishes, Leslie ate boxed noodles—fettuccine Alfredo or shells and cheese. Leslie also drank very little water. Consequentially, she emptied her bowels every two to three days—a routine she didn't know, until recently, was unusual or unhealthy.

"I learned from Molly to eat from the perimeter of the store—REAL food!" Leslie explains, "I counted my five fruits and vegetables a day. And I started drinking half my weight in water, roughly 60 ounces a day." With this increased fiber and hydration, Leslie's bathroom habits got much more regular, so that she "went" two times a day. Her pain, itching and inflammation disappeared.

Leslie notes, "Doctors always told me to eat more fiber and drink more water, but none of them gave me *specifics*. I grew up not knowing how to eat properly. So I never really knew that I had to overhaul my diet." The 21-Day Action Plan gave Leslie "specific, measurable goals" as well as recipes and replacements for the processed foods she needed to give up. Leslie also reveals, "Unlike other weight-focused diet plans, your program, Molly, is about healthy, *vibrant living*."

Now Leslie eats five small meals a day, starting her day with a cup of Fiber One® cereal and fresh berries and vanilla Greek yogurt she brings with her to work. "I had never eaten blackberries before. I love alternating

GET THE LOWDOWN ON PORTIONS

Serving sizes can be daunting if you've never paid attention to how much you're eating. But establishing reasonable portions is essential for weight management and good nutrition. Here are a few simple guidelines to follow, and be sure to use the *Grocery List* (page 82) for suggestions.

Vegetables:

- Eat a minimum of three or four 1-cup servings daily and make sure to consume a variety of vibrantly colored vegetables (dark green, yellow, orange and red) every day.
- Include at least one cup of spinach or kale daily, as they are powerhouse foods high in vitamins A, C and K.
- Vegetables like broccoli and peppers also help to balance blood sugar, preventing us from overeating while helping to reduce blood pressure and the risk of heart disease, stroke and some cancers.
- Eat white-flesh vegetables like cauliflower and cucumbers, as they may protect against stroke.
- Limit your intake of starchy vegetables such as potatoes, peas and corn to a one-half cup serving and eat them occasionally, not daily.

Fruit:

- Eat a variety of two or three 1-cup servings daily. A half of a banana, a third of an avocado, a whole apple, orange, plum, etc. and one quarter-cup of dried fruit are each considered a serving. If you don't have a measuring cup, a good rule to follow is to allow yourself a palm-sized portion of whatever it is you're eating.
- Fruits are rich in vitamins A and C and folate. Other essential nutrients, antioxidants, and fiber can help guard against heart disease and stroke, some types of cancer and vision loss.
- White-flesh fruits such as pears, bananas and apples also prevent stroke. One apple a day is a great way to increase white fruit intake.[23]

Whole Grains:

- One slice of whole grain or rye bread
- A half-cup of brown rice, barley or quinoa (also a complete protein source)
- A three-quarter cup of high fiber, whole grain cereal
- One whole grain English muffin
- A cup of cooked high fiber or whole grain pasta
- A half-cup of Old-Fashioned, plain oats

(Continued on the next page)

GET THE LOWDOWN ON PORTIONS *(Continued from page 35)*

Proteins:

- Beans and legumes are a major source of complex carbohydrates, fiber, protein, calcium, zinc, iron and folate. A half-cup serving can be added to soup, sauce, brown rice, quinoa or salads or it can be enjoyed as a side dish.
- When eating lean meat (white is best) or fish, 3 ounces (the size of a deck of cards) is considered to be one serving.
- Nuts, especially unsalted almonds (technically seeds), walnuts, cashews, pistachios and Brazil nuts, are a terrific source of "good" fats, fiber, protein and antioxidants. But because they are high in calories, limit yourself to a serving size of 12 to 15. Add them to smoothies, salads, yogurt and cereal or eat them as a snack between meals. A tablespoon (about the size of a Ping-Pong ball) of pumpkin, flax or chia seeds is also a good option.
- Eggs are one of the least expensive forms of protein, and the American Heart Association says most adults can safely eat one or two per day.

Fats:

- Make extra virgin olive oil, coconut oil or 100 percent avocado oil your fat of choice. A 1-tablespoon serving can be used for sautéing or drizzled on vegetables and salad for extra flavor. All three oils are high in monounsaturated fat, the healthy dietary fat your body needs to balance cholesterol levels, and all are rich in antioxidants. They help lower the risk of heart disease by reducing risk factors and can also help satisfy your appetite.
- Avocado oil may not be as well known as olive oil, but it is high in vitamins A, D and E. Avocados have more protein than any other fruit and more potassium than a banana. Avocado oil has a velvety, buttery texture and has the highest smoke point (450 degrees) of all plant oils.
- Butter, on the other hand, should be used sparingly; about 1 tablespoon of unsalted butter per day is reasonable. Avoid margarine and fried foods.

Dairy:

- A cup of 1 percent organic milk (I prefer it over skim milk because the fat makes it more filling)
- An ounce (or the size of a pair of dice) of low/reduced-fat cheese
- Small container of Greek yogurt
- A half-cup cottage cheese
- These foods are excellent sources of protein, they contain calcium and some are fortified with vitamin D to promote strong bones and teeth and prevent osteoporosis.
- With all the above, *read labels and follow the serving size recommendations on the package.*

between them—the raspberries, blackberries and strawberries." For lunch, she often brought wraps with beans, mango and salsa.

In this way, Leslie exclaims, "I have taken control of my body." Now she says, "My life is better in so many ways. There's now a man in my life, and I'm enjoying cooking for us, roasting vegetables and expanding our healthy menus." She went on to say, "This is the best I have ever felt. I am *only* drinking water (except for the occasional glass of wine), and I have learned to live vibrantly. You have changed my life forever!"

Just like it did for Leslie, eating REAL will engage you in ways you never anticipated—so that you try strange and wonderful new recipes, combinations of foods, and regional cuisines. You may discover the kitchen to be the perfect setting for bonding with friends or a new companion.

EAT REAL, BE REAL

When real food gets into your body, literally into your DNA, it changes you. For me, down-to-earth eating is a part of a connected life, staying rooted in the values of my upbringing.

I grew up in Kittanning, a small town in Pennsylvania, with three stop lights and a Dairy Queen. There I hung out in my mom's beauty shop where I loved to remove the "curlies," or rollers, for the sweet ladies who came to the salon. Though my parents were not sure why I felt the need—given that I was expected to take over the salon or the family gas station—I was the first person in my family to go to and graduate from college.

Fast forward 30 years and I live an urban life, full of culture, bustle, people and distraction. Today I have the means to eat out frequently or maybe even hire a chef, but that has never been a desire of mine. I'd much rather cook and bake at home in the evenings with my family and friends, even after full days of work and driving my children to their daily, after-school activities. When I do go out, I thoroughly enjoy *the treat* that it is.

For me, eating real is also about being real, and modeling real living for my children and the clients I help. I'm not interested in plastic surgery, Botox or $400 face creams. I don't get my teeth whitened. (Well, I did try it once when I made the Ravens cheerleading squad—but the gel fried my gums.) I stick to the whitening toothpastes, such as Crest Pro-Health™ and Colgate™ Optic White. Keeping it real, none of the photos in this book are airbrushed or Photoshopped.

I think many of us can benefit from asking ourselves: in what ways am I not living a real and grounded life? Where have I allowed convenience to supersede health?

Many of us will think nothing of spending $4 on a box of chemical-laden cookies but resist a piece of vitamin-loaded, organic fruit we perceive to be too expensive. We fail to *pause, think and act*. Instead, we rush, ignore and hit the drive-through.

It is an intentional act to say thanks for the food in front of us and do more to ensure that everyone around us has a place at the table. Truly, we grow healthier when we stay attuned to the gifts God has given us, and become less impressed with human concoctions and window dressings.

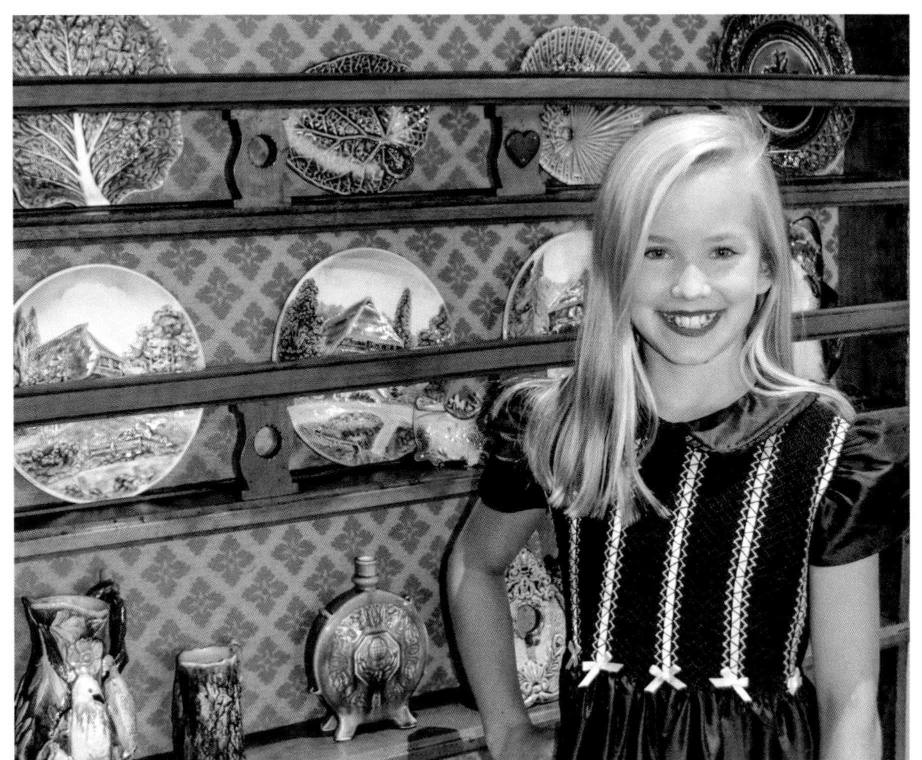

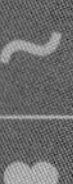

My daughter, Lillian, next to Majolica pottery which has been passed down in my family for generations. We used a variety of these pieces to shoot the food images in this book because they are so special to me. Identify or create family traditions and find ways to make them a part of your life.

EMOTIONAL EATING

Pause for water before you eat. Pause before your meal to say grace. Then pause again, if you're having a bad day and are about to inhale a New York cheesecake. Might you be using food as salve for an emotional wound?

I'm going to level with you. There is one time of the month when I have to have a heaping serving of French fries—with every last fry dipped in mayonnaise and ketchup. I follow that up with *an entire slice* of lava cake. Sometimes even another three bites of lemon cake to top it off. I don't deny myself when hormones hit. I just know that they will soon pass.

I do keep a stash of chocolate in my house at all times. Otherwise I rip into the chocolate chips bag, and they spill everywhere, and I find little nibs of chocolate in my cabinets for the next three weeks. If there is no

PLAN TO EAT REAL

Be grateful. Be connected. Eat REAL. It all starts with your taking control of your eating!

You can do this by getting organized and gaining a understanding of appropriate serving sizes. Review the *Grocery List* (page 82). Let the suggestions guide your meal planning and snacks to ensure you have wholesome food easily available to you throughout the day.

Three REAL Meals

Breakfast is the most important meal of the day because it awakens your metabolism.

Start by eating fruit first thing in the morning. I especially love strawberries, blueberries, raspberries, grapefruits, oranges and cantaloupes because they are loaded with vitamin C, fiber, calcium and folic acid. All of these vitamins and minerals are absolutely necessary for sustained good health. Fruit is a great choice any time of day, and because it's easy to digest, I eat it before anything else so it's not sitting on top of foods that take longer to absorb into my system.

Add variety to your breakfast routine throughout the week to ensure you're beginning each day with a range of nourishment, nutrition, flavor and texture.

Lunch should be under your control, even when you are on-the-go. If you're away from home during the day, plan ahead and pack your lunch and snacks. When you're hungry and have no healthy options, you're more likely to eat empty calories, more "bad" fat and processed food.

The night before work, school or a full day of errands, prepare a lunch that includes fruit, vegetables and a protein as well as a snack.

Celery sticks with 1 tablespoon of peanut butter, hard-boiled eggs, raw vegetables, fresh fruit and unsalted almonds and walnuts are good munchies. The best combination for filling you up is pairing a protein with a carbohydrate (for instance, a small apple with a slice of reduced-fat cheese).

If you're eating a sandwich for lunch, eat only one slice of whole grain bread or replace it with spinach or a thick slice of tomato. Add half a slice of cheese broken into chunks to trick your mind into thinking it's a full serving. Use only reduced-fat or light mayonnaise or skip it and add Dijon mustard for a lower calorie flavor option.

Dinner is a time to make sure you get the vegetables your body needs. Make it a practice to fill two-thirds of your plate at dinner with a variety of vegetables so that you're proactively filling up on what's good for you.

PLAN TO EAT REAL *(Continued from page 39)*

How & When

Eat Mindfully. Chew slowly (15 times or more with every forkful), putting your utensil down after a few bites of food, so you can savor every morsel while dining in a peaceful environment free of television and bright lights. This is a wonderful way to de-stress after a busy day. And, as an important bonus, studies have shown people consume fewer calories in this type of environment.[24]

Eat early. Make it a practice to finish dinner by 6:30 p.m. on most nights of the week. I believe it's healthier to allow your food to digest before bed, and then you'll have time for a walk or some other light exercise that may help you sleep more soundly.

Strive for balance

Take advantage of the *Make REAL Meals* I am sharing (pages 148–175) as part of your program to get healthy. You'll find you can cook delicious, nutritious food without a lot of fuss or exotic ingredients.

Set yourself up for healthier eating by planning for the entire week including breakfast, lunch, dinner and snacks. That way you'll be sure to get the essential daily dose of the vitamins, carbohydrates, proteins, fiber, whole grains and fats your body needs to perform at its peak. If you are eating a balanced diet that includes a large variety of fruits and vegetables, you will naturally get the range of nutrients required for good health. But you should check with your physician to make sure you don't have a medical condition that requires specific supplements.

The *Make REAL Meals* section also includes basic suggestions for breakfast, lunch, dinner, snacks and desserts. So even if you're not a cook and do not plan on becoming one, you will have a better sense of what you should be eating throughout each day.

A few words about sweets

Sweets should be eaten only as a treat. Take your sweet intake seriously—too often, we consume more calories and fat through sweets than through the nutritious food our bodies require for optimal health.

Are you one of those people, like me, who always wants something sweet after a meal in order to feel satisfied? This craving is a result of habit and association. To break it, you either need to change up your routine after meals or set a strict rule about how much you're going to eat. For example, make it routine to immediately leave the kitchen/dining room and go for a walk after your meal. Choose fresh fruit for dessert or limit yourself to one homemade cookie, not four. Bake treats and freeze them in single servings. Deprivation is not the answer because it can set you up for wild cravings or binges.

I suggest you enjoy sweet pleasures, but do so in moderation. One serving of whatever it is, period!

higher quality chocolate in the house, I will turn the house upside down, looking for the chocolate Easter bunny one of my kids ate the head off and then forgot about. By the way, if you dunk the decapitated bunny into peanut butter, it actually hides the white age marks the chocolate acquires over months of laying in hiding.

All of us have times in our lives when we resort to emotional eating. Yes, even me, Susie Cheerleader, the one in high school you loved to hate because I was blonde and bubbly. I've faced some hardships. In my journey to become a mom, I miscarried six times. With all three of my children, I cried buckets of tears when each one was born with breathing problems and had to spend time in a neonatal intensive care unit. It's devastating to lose a close friend to brain cancer and another to a horrific accident. And it's devastating to separate from my husband and best friend, to let go of the dream for our marriage after 17 years.

But in life, we have control over how long it impairs our ability to function normally. We have a modicum of control over how much emotional eating we allow ourselves.

We can grieve without allowing sadness and self-defeating habits to compromise our energy and cripple our health.

YOU ARE IN CONTROL, YOU ARE CONNECTED

Forgive yourself today. Tomorrow, move on. When chaos hits, focus on what you can do personally to alleviate the situation. Or try to find the opportunity to learn or grow from the muck you are in. Don't let the ebb and flow of life eat away at your health and energy.

Pause. Think. Act. *Move away from the cheesecake.* Go for a walk. Get some fresh air. Engage with the natural world. Breathe in through your nose slowly, deep into your belly, and blow the air out through your mouth. And take 12 big gulps of *water*.

Michael Pollan writes, "The way we eat represents our most profound engagement with the natural world. Daily, our eating turns nature into culture, transforming the body of the world into our bodies and minds."[25]

For me, the tenet of eating real is one of connection and gratitude. When I am grateful, I feel grounded. When I say grace, I get clear on my place in the universe, on the fact that life doesn't revolve around me. I am made from the earth and I was placed here on earth to serve. My delight comes from serving God, honoring my body with food of the earth and honoring others with all of my gifts.

What do you have for which you are grateful? How are you connected to this beautiful planet, its resources and to other human beings? Whom does God want you to invite to your table? Foster these beautiful and meaning-filled ties with love made manifest, a diet rich with nutrients and with clear intentions for your health.

Exercise Daily

A MESSAGE OF DISCIPLINE & FAITH

"A bear, however hard he tries, grows tubby without exercise."
—A.A. *Milne*

Five years ago, I was washing my son Wyatt's hair in the tub when a feeling came over me that something was terribly wrong. I ran my fingers over a large bump on his scalp that his pediatrician had, for five years, told me was nothing. "His head was just growing," the first doctor had said, as well as the second opinion. But that night, I became certain this bulge on Wyatt's skull was not normal, and that God was pressing me to pursue more answers.

Within days, seven-year-old Wyatt was scheduled for an MRI, a procedure we were told would last about 20 minutes. An hour and 40 minutes later, a neurologist brought my sweet, baby-faced boy into an exam room where his father and I were waiting. The doctor began to tell us the news that somewhere in my heart, I already knew.

"Your son has a very large mass on his brain, a size we have never seen before in a child his . . ." the doctor began.

I was, in that moment, no longer in my body. The way that I remember it, I was looking down on the four of us in the room—my husband, my son, the doctor and myself.

Before the neurologist could continue, I raised my hand, my pointer finger extending up as if to say: One moment. Give me a moment. Just *stop*.

I then rushed out of the room, down the hall, and fell on my knees, sobbing. I don't remember much of it, except that within a moment or two, I got back up. I found a nurse and insisted that Wyatt be removed from the room and distracted with a story about where he had traveled that summer. I was crystal clear on one thing—that Wyatt be sheltered from news that would only be confusing or scary to him.

Pause. Think. Act.

Wyatt, we learned, had an arachnoid cyst, a benign growth of a size that was very unusual.

The growth took up nearly 40 percent of his brain space rather than 1 percent, as is typical of this rare condition. His skull was, as a result, paper thin from the presence and pressure of this hard tumor, and this made him vulnerable to seizures, strokes and irreversible damage to his eye sight, hearing, speech and behavior. Of course, Wyatt was also in danger because any blow to his head, so common in the rough and tumble world of seven-year-old boys, could be life threatening.

For the next several weeks, we met with neurosurgeons across the country about Wyatt's condition and he went on to have surgery—in which holes were intricately created in the deep cisterns of his brain, allowing the fluid in the cyst to circulate and for the balloon, as we explained the cyst to him, to become less taut. The surgeons put several hundred titanium screws in Wyatt's head when they closed his skull. There were no guarantees, the doctors said, but the surgery had gone well.

Wyatt is now 12 years old, in 7th grade and he's a "straight A" student—well, he'd beg to differ because he did get a B+ last year. There are no residual learning differences or behavioral challenges. With a reinforced helmet, Wyatt runs and plays, hikes and throws. He plays lacrosse and soccer, all of it with a zeal, determination and a bright smile on his face. Every day with Wyatt is a gift we delight in, and feel so lucky to get.

I tell you this story for two reasons. One, it has an incredibly happy ending, despite starting out in a place of enormous fear and uncertainty. Two, it demonstrates the power of pause, think and act. Because in the scariest moment I can ever imagine having, my instinct was to stop the doctor from saying any more. I knew enough to point my finger in the air, as if to say, "No, I'm sorry, this is not my truth. This is not Wyatt's truth. Our truth comes from God and God alone."

To this day, I have never "googled" Wyatt's medical condition. Nor have I spent hours poring over the possible complications of the large mass that remains in his head. I honestly believe we pollute our minds with too much information these days, and I didn't want to know more. With medicine, I was already clear, there is so much more unknown than there is known.

It starts with the pause, taking a moment to reassert the source of your strength and protection. It continues with thought—in my case, on my knees, surrendering and asking for guidance. Then swiftly, I was moved to act, clear that my first priority was to get my son safe from too much information—from words that could be unsettling.

Ultimately, we chose as a family to focus on the good—to put into perspective the fact that the situation could have been far worse—and to devote ourselves to enjoying every minute we spent together.

THE GIFT OF EACH DAY

Truly, I believe, our family got through this crisis in large part because we were very healthy. Wyatt was, in every sense, a healthy boy, so that he was an ideal candidate for a very difficult and risky surgery. I was able to stay focused on Wyatt and the rest of my family, without descending into depression or a paralysis of fear, because I was mentally and physically sharp.

For us, fitness is how we live out our faith. We believe that we are better equipped to respond to all the tests and challenges of life because we attend regularly to the health with which we are endowed. We are not sitting idly, waiting for life to happen to us. We choose to move.

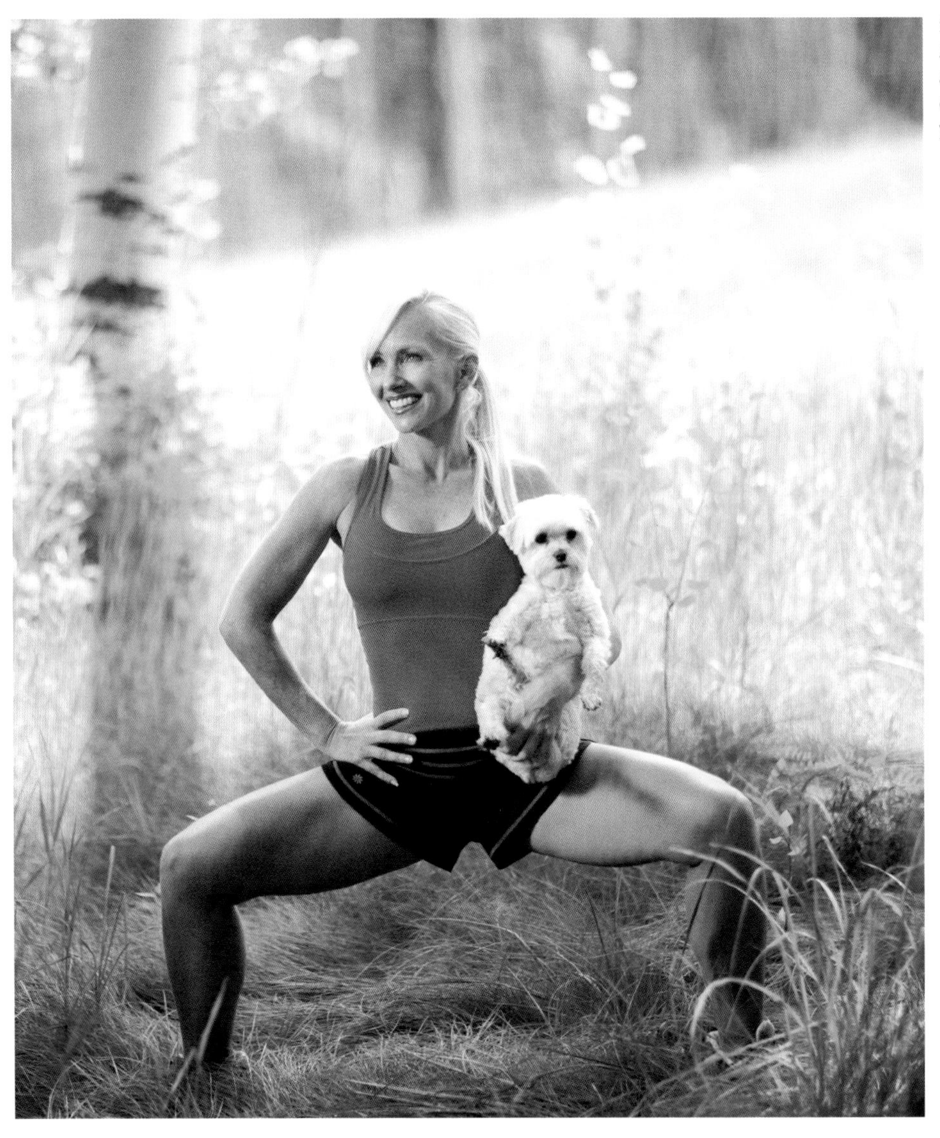

Slot exercise in your schedule, 30 minutes every day. Have a Plan A, then a Plan B, in case life tries to intervene with your healthy habit.

Less than a fifth of American adults get the recommended amount of exercise each week, and more than a quarter of us get none at all. We *know* it's good for us. But every week, we allow our work, family, household and leisure activities to supersede our body's basic need—*to move*.

Daily exercise is the third pillar because it transforms your fitness, your energy level and your mood.

You lose weight, you sleep better and it helps you stave off heart disease, diabetes and a slew of other medical problems. You look better, you feel sexier, and once you start exercising—and overcome the inertia—it gets easier to do it again.

Woody Allen said that "90 percent of success is showing up." And, every day, you show up at work, at your kids' carpool, at your friend's birthday lunch, at the school bake sale or the band performance, at the pharmacy to pick up your dad's prescription, and at your big screen for Monday Night Football. When will it be time for you to show up . . . *for you*?

IS IT OVER YET?

I'm not going to ask you to get out of bed at the crack of dawn to go to a gym or a boot camp. I am certainly not an early morning person. I get up at 6:45 AM and until I guzzle my first 30 ounces of water, I am foggy and tired. For me, the best time to exercise is in the afternoons—right before I pick up my kids—because I'm headed into three hours of driving around in my SUV and getting them to practices and activities. Though there's no proof, I suspect that the more we sit, the wider our butts get. So I try to limit and counteract the tush time!

For me, the second best time for me to exercise in the evenings. I do the push-up and leg routine with my kids. Or after they are asleep, I get down to cardio. For nearly 30 years, I've built into my day a half-hour or more of leg lifts, squats, kicks and cardio-dance, the moves of which are included in your 21-Day Action Plan. That's how I maintain my weight, *doing just 30 minutes of exercise each day*, along with drinking water and being thoughtful about the food I put in my mouth.

So I am asking you to make the same 30-minute commitment, to look at your day and figure out when you can fit in a half-hour for yourself.

If a morning meeting means all you can fit in is a 10-minute walk, then by all means, go for 10 minutes and hit the pavement again for 20 minutes after dinner. Have a Plan A and a Plan B. But slot 30 minutes in somehow!

Exercising your way—whether with walking, running, yoga or the elliptical—for 30 minutes a day, you will exceed the Center for Disease Control's recommended 150 minutes a week.[26] In keeping with the guidelines, do full-body strength training for two or three of your weekly workouts. And you *will* change your life, from the inside out.

WOW, WHAT RESULTS!

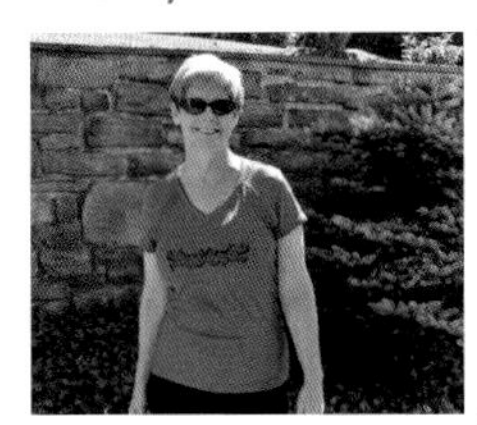

Karen
AGE 57
OCCUPATION Life Coach and Consultant
HOMETOWN Forest Hill, MD

Fifty-seven-year-old life coach and consultant Karen has gone in cycles all her life, sometimes quite active and other times, going months without working out. "Most days, I put it off, letting everything else come before exercise. By the time evening rolled around, I got tired and my motivation was gone." In October 2012, she joined one of my 21-Day Action groups to kick-start her weight loss and fitness.

Karen began the plan by drinking 90 ounces of water a day, applying the first pillar to her health. Immediately, Karen, a chronic migraine sufferer, noticed her headaches were dissipating, or not coming on at all. Check, she incorporated the second pillar, too, adding more fruit and vegetables to her diet. Karen entered everything she ate in the 21-Day journal, even on nights when she had to write "Too many chips!"

For a bi-weekly dose of adrenaline, Karen attended exercise classes I led with her 21-Day group. "At first," Karen says, "I could do maybe one regular push-up, perhaps a few more on my knees." Within the first week, Karen lost 4 pounds so her motivation to work out—first at a lower intensity, then gradually increasing—grew strong. In time, Karen could do the 100 push-ups in intervals on the Molly Vibrant Living DVD—75 percent of them plank-style, the rest on her knees.

On days when exercise was tough to squeeze in, Karen followed the 21-Day Action Plan advice. "Just walk for 10 minutes in the morning and 20 later on," she said, beginning to think ahead and *plan her workouts*. In seven months, Karen lost 29 pounds, dropping from a size 16 to a size 8 or 10 (depending on the brand) and losing 29 inches from her waist, tummy, bottom and thighs. Her blood pressure, which was nearing the point of requiring medication, dropped within normal range in the first three months.

"Seeing those results is . . . wow!" Karen smiles, "People tell me all the time how much healthier I look, not just my body, but my skin—brighter and younger."

THE UNCANNY DIFFERENCE EXERCISE MAKES

As Karen discovered, 30 minutes of daily exercise—especially combined with great hydration and nutrition—provides a wowing makeover. Here's six uncanny ways workouts change your physiology:

Boost Your Heart. Aerobic exercise strengthens your heart and can lower blood pressure by increasing blood circulation throughout your beautiful body.

- Exercise actually increases your good HDL cholesterol so that it can give the heave-ho to the bad LDL cholesterol lining the walls of your blood vessels, sending it back to the liver for re-processing.[27] Bye bye, bad cholesterol.
- Regular exercise can decrease your risk for a heart attack by making the heart more efficient at delivering oxygen to all parts of the body. That's part of the reason you *feel better* after exercising.

UNDERSTANDING YOUR BMR[28]

You burn calories while you are active and at rest. Your body needs a certain number of calories for breathing, cell growth, regulating body temperature, blood circulation, brain and nerve function and other physiological processes. The amount of calories you need for these basic functions is called your Basal Metabolic Rate (BMR).It accounts for 60 to 75 percent of the calories you burn every day and is influenced by several factors, namely:

1) **Body Composition:** The more muscle you have, the higher your metabolic rate tends to be since muscle burns 3-5 times more calories than fat does.

2) **Age:** Metabolic rate is highest during periods of rapid growth. As you get older, muscle decreases and metabolism naturally slows—about 2-5% per decade after age 40.

3) **Weight:** The heavier you are, the more calories you need. This is a key reason why it's easier to lose weight at the start of a diet and more difficult later.

4) **Gender:** Women, in general, have a lower metabolic rate than men because men naturally have more muscle.

5) **Body Surface Area:** The greater your body's skin area, the higher your BMR. Tall people tend to have higher BMRs.

6) **Endocrine Glands:** Thyroid hormones are the principal regulators of metabolic rate.

In addition, if the body perceives starvation, a person's metabolic rate can drop as much as 50 percent below normal. The human body is programmed for survival and interprets big reductions in calories as starvation. This, in turn, prompts all systems to conserve energy and is the overriding reason extreme calorie restriction ("starvation diets") never succeeds.

The best way to determine how many calories you need to function each day is to use a BMR calculator. The BMR calculator is based on your height, weight, age, gender and level of physical weekly activity. You can find one online to determine your BMR. Remember, this formula isn't exact because of muscle mass versus fat ratio and other contributing factors. I do not recommend that you count calories because it puts too much emphasis on food—not enough on the other factors.

SLEEP SOUNDLY

As I mentioned earlier, exercise promotes better sleep. And a good night's sleep provides the energy you need to pursue your fitness goals. Get a peaceful night of rest, as you...

- **Begin clearing your mind before bed.** Move away from your laptop, mobile device, tablet and TV at least one hour before you lay your head down on your pillow.
- **Keep your phone out of your bedroom.** It's too tempting to check messages and the dinging and flashing all night long disrupts your sleep. Don't affect the sleep of a loved one in the "real world" while you spend time on your devices. Besides, a number of studies suggest that cell phone radiation may be linked to brain cancer.[29] Nothing is conclusive, but why take the chance when you most certainly don't need your phone nearby when you are sleeping?
- **Improve air circulation.** Use a humidifier or crack open a window.
- **Keep a pen and small notebook or pad of paper beside your bed.** Write down any "to do" tasks for the next day or ideas you would like to pursue. Putting thoughts to paper is a productive way to clear your head for restful sleep. I've used this technique for years and it keeps me sane and organized.
- **Wake up at the same time every day.** Your internal biological clock craves consistency. The more you stick to a schedule, the easier it is for you to fall asleep and wake up.
- **Relax naturally.** Take a bubble bath and add lavender. Listen to slow, steady music such as classical, Celtic, or New Age.
- **Limit your fluid intake** at least an hour prior to bedtime and avoid caffeine, especially in the evening.
- **Use all-natural bedding and sleepwear** to maintain your normal body temperature.
- **Pray.** Each day, remind yourself or share with family and friends the things for which you are grateful. Pray for others in need.
- **Read inspiring quotes** for a few minutes then turn out your light.
- **Stretch your arms, legs, back and neck** before turning off the light.
- **Create your own bedtime routine** to train your body that it's time to sleep.

Boost Your Metabolism. Bottom line, you burn calories when you *move*. Your metabolism's job is to convert the food you eat into fuel. But when you overeat and you don't exercise, your metabolism has no choice but to store the fat for you, usually in places where everyone can see it!

- By exercising regularly and consistently, you burn more calories and prevent excess calories from being stored as fat. Over time, you shed fat that was already put on the shelf!
- Strength training and weight lifting also changes your resting metabolic rate, so that your body burns calories even when you are not exercising.[30] With weight training done, you take a nap and still burn off some of a burrito. Imagine that!

Boost Your Bone Mass. Resistance training exercises such as push-ups, weight lifting, pull-ups, biking, rowing, swimming and even walking help preserve bone mass, increase bone density, and strengthen muscles.[31]

- Without physical activity, the vitamins you take to combat osteoporosis—a condition most of us get when we are 70 years or older—are nearly useless.
- Moderate weight-bearing exercises such as walking, along with specific strength training such as push-ups, squats, lunges and swimming can help *restore* calcium—which we lose as we age, and in osteoporosis—and, in turn, strengthens our bones.

Boost Your Sleep. Exercise can improve quality of sleep, especially a few hours before bedtime.

- Regular aerobic exercise and stretching makes it easier to fall asleep at night and keep snoozing longer.[32]
- Numerous studies report the relationship between insufficient sleep and weight gain.[33] Aim for seven to eight hours of sack time each night—to whittle your waistline and to have sweet dreams.

Boost Your Mood. You are so much nicer of a person when you exercise, am I right? Physical activity can be a powerful mood enhancer.[34]

- Exercise stimulates the production of endorphins—neurotransmitters that produce feelings of well-being.
- Exercise provides "natural" pain relief and can help you relax and fend off depression.
- When you drop some pounds, you feel great. It bolsters your confidence and you enjoy more compliments. Your mood is decidedly improved!

Boost Your Chemistry. Staying physically active detoxifies your body.

- Physical movement improves the functioning of the lymphatic system, which carries nutrients to cells in your body and then carries waste products away. This process helps clear away infection and keeps body fluids in balance.
- Exercise also boosts sex drive, making you more easily aroused, and combating stress—one of the big inhibitors of libido.[35] When you get a bit more svelte, va-va voom is much more appealing.

To reap these marvelous effects, however, *you need to be consistent*. You need to show up for 30 minutes or more every day. Do it for yourself and the future you—yes, you, child of God—richly deserve to enjoy.

You do need to show up for God, who designed your brilliant body to benefit from play and movement. Prayer, after all, isn't meant only to be something we do sitting down. For thousands of years, believers have embarked on prayer walks and pilgrimages, epic journeys to Lourdes, Mecca and other endpoints with sacred and healing power. As disciples do, they allow themselves to be led far outside their comfort zones, to spiritual destinations of immense meaning and power. Being outdoors, moving our bodies, we can also pursue our lives' higher purpose.

Try this tonight: Go outside on a walk without ear buds. Fill your chest with fresh air and be grateful for the gift of this day, for the soft grass and fragrant flowers, as well as the gifts of your body. Focus on the sound of your footfall, the rhythmic pattern of your feet on the sidewalk or in the grass. In prayer, we talk to God, but in meditative moments such as these, we *listen* to God. Like the disciples, allow yourself to be guided on a journey not of your own design.

GETTING STARTED AND STAYING DISCIPLINED

How can you be a disciple—someone who is faithful to your God-given body, calling forth all its potential for health and goodness in the world? Having helped many people make enduring changes in their fitness and energy, I've found that three key factors buttress a new exercise routine and help you sustain your workout habit:

Consistency

How do you persuade yourself to keep *showing up* for exercise, day after day? Let's break it down:

1. Pace Yourself. Whether you take a group fitness class, follow an exercise DVD (such as the The Vibrant Living Workout), or participate in another form of exercise, never force yourself to go beyond your personal limits. Don't overdo the first day and never come back!
   - Stop exercising if you feel strain or pain, have difficulty breathing, or experience dizziness or a sudden drain of energy.
   - If you haven't exercised for a long period of time, start with 10 to 15 minutes a day for the first week and increase your activity by five minutes a day each week thereafter until you are comfortably exercising at least 30 minutes daily. Included with the 21-Day Action Plan is a suggested weekly exercise plan (see pages 93, 109, and 125). Follow it to learn how to move your body, strengthen your core, increase lean muscle tissue and become the physically fit person you want to be.
2. Make more moves. Incorporate bits of movement into your life whenever you can. One of the most effective ways to increase your physical activity is to wear a pedometer. The American Heart Association recommends people walk 10,000 steps in the course of a day to help reduce body mass index (BMI) and lower blood pressure. This may seem like a lot of stepping, but just like NIKE™ says, Just Do It! Start now and be sure to check your pedometer throughout the day, as you'll know by noon if you need to get off your tush.

- Take the stairs two at a time, mow your lawn, park in a spot the farthest distance from the door, ride a bike instead of driving when possible and walk to give a person a message at your office instead of sending an email.
- On each day of your 21-Day Action Plan, you'll find an easy-to-follow *Knock-Out Move of the Day* to learn and do frequently to help tone and strengthen your body. These moves can be combined to create a complete workout that you can do anywhere, anytime.

- Running is a great cardiovascular workout, but walking is equally beneficial. So if you are one of the many people who find it difficult to run or jog for any distance, take heart. A 30-minute brisk walk mixed with short sprints every four minutes is even more beneficial than 40 minutes of running. Numerous studies show that interval training is more effective than steady jogging. In fact, those who did a walk-run instead of a steady jog lost three times the fat from their legs and butt, according to a study from University of New South Wales in Sydney.[36]
- Never run outdoors with music in your ears. Enjoy the sounds of nature and protect yourself by being aware of your surroundings. Too many people are attacked when jogging, speaking from personal experience. Fortunately, when someone tried to do it to me, I wasn't wearing headphones—which saved me.
- Record your steps in the Exercise box in the *Daily Log* to keep on track. Go to www.mollyshattuck.com to find out what pedometers we recommend and offer.

3. **Feel your muscle.** Enjoy seeing your body change as you build muscle and as your body becomes firmer, stronger and more flexible. Muscle and fat weigh precisely the same, but fat occupies more space and muscle is denser. Having a higher ratio of muscle speeds up your metabolism and promotes a greater calorie burn, even while you're resting. So, congratulate yourself. Show off your guns. Your added muscle is an essential component of overall fat loss.

4. **Look the part.** Work out in breathable athletic attire. Studies have shown that people are more serious about whatever they are doing if they "dress the part." I also have found that wearing clothes that fit helps with form when exercising. We are more

VARY YOUR MOVES

Here are ideas to get physical and do more in the great outdoors:

- Bike
- Dance to your favorite music!
- Hike
- Jog
- Jump rope
- Paddle board
- Racquetball
- Rock climb
- Rollerblade
- Squash
- Snowshoe
- Ski
- Swim
- Throw a football with kids or friends
- Tennis
- Walk-Run combination

EXERCISE YOUR BRAIN

Being mentally fit is as important as being physically fit. Exercising your brain may deter the age-related, cognitive decline associated with degenerative diseases like Alzheimer's and dementia. Critical thinking stimulates brain cells and, in some cases, can grow new brain pathways. After dinner with my kids, I love to do brain-teaser exercises (e.g., Sudoku, crossword puzzles, Lumosity.com, and other games) for 15 to 20 minutes. I am convinced Sudoku helps me think more clearly.

More Brain Push-ups

Forcing your brain to think about alternative ways of doing ordinary tasks can awaken the idea of living more curiously and intentionally. Include these brain push-ups in your daily routine:

- Use your non-dominant hand to brush your teeth.
- Try alternative routes to school, work, grocery store, etc.
- Log on to your computer with your opposite hand.
- Get dressed or showered with your eyes closed.
- Brush your teeth while standing on one leg.
- Link activities with smells. For instance, light a candle and listen to classical music while relaxing in the tub. Smell a garlic clove or fresh lemon when walking through the kitchen.
- Vary the order of your "get ready for the day" routine and activities. But remember to begin drinking water as soon as wake up—and throughout the day.
- Take different routes to walk the dog, drive to work, pick up kids from school and run regular errands.

All of this variety will lead you in the direction of wanting more in your life as it opens your brain to curious thinking and living *intentionally*. That's what it has done for me, and I love the adventure.

conscientious of our posture and tend to hold in our bellies, and that's great for the core!

5. **Take it in.** Buy a full-length mirror if you don't have one, so you can become more aware of the way you are doing push-ups, dance moves and lunges and so you can observe your posture. Consider the mirror a check system for doing the moves correctly. Regardless of what exercise you're doing, good posture equates to more use of your core (belly) muscles. Furthermore, poor posture contributes to chronic back and neck pain and can drain your energy.

6. **Eat dinner early.** Try to finish dinner by 6:30 p.m. when possible. This way your food has time to digest before you do push-ups, squats, lunges, jumping jacks or any other exercises while watching television or listening to music before bedtime. Even if you're not planning on moving your body at night, most people will find that easier digestion and

sounder sleep can be achieved by *not* consuming a heavy meal right before going to bed.

7. **Don't overeat.** Don't fall into the trap of letting exercise become an excuse for overeating. The calories burned from different activities vary based on weight, age and gender. To burn the calories from a few minutes of super-sized snacking, you would have to exercise intensely for another several hours.

Variety

Find physical activities you like such as jumping on a trampoline, bicycling and dancing, and do them often at varying degrees of intensity. Never do the same exercise two days in row, because you can over-stress a particular muscle group. It's best to mix up your routine and alternate between cardio and strength training. Furthermore, your body responds to bursts of new moves. If you run every day, your body becomes accustomed to it—and doesn't burn as much energy. When you change up your routine, you burn more calories and you avoid repetition and boredom.

When I ran the Marine Corps Marathon in 1997, I trained by running three nonconsecutive days per week (two shorter runs and one longer one) and did other cardio workouts like rollerblading, swimming and dancing, along with push-ups and leg lifts, on the days in between. My longest run was 16.5 miles and yet I was able to run the entire 26.2 at my pace of 10-minute miles—exactly how I had trained. It worked because I wasn't overusing the same muscles day in and day out for months on end. Be sure to follow the *Weekly Exercise Schedules* I have provided on pages 93, 109 and 125, along with the daily *Knock-Out Move of the Day* exercises featured in your *Daily Log*.

Planning and Compartmentalizing

Now that we've anticipated the things your body needs to be consistent with exercise, let's attend to your mind and soul. How can you outmaneuver the reluctant mind or the weary spirit?

1. **Schedule your workouts.** You'll find an *Exercise Schedule* in the **21-Day Action Plan** so you can make appointments with yourself.
    - Consider them holy, these times you have set to transform your body and your life.
    - If you can't squeeze in a half hour, go for 15 minutes. But keep the daily routine so that it becomes a treasured ritual in your life.
    - Don't dismiss the importance of daily choices. Be aware of all the ways you can infuse your body with health, strength and energy—with water, with real food and with daily exercise.

    Kent Nerburn, the author of *Small Graces: The Quiet Gifts of Everyday Life*, writes, "Ritual is routine infused with mindfulness. It is habit made holy." Having spent six months living in a monastic community, he says:

    "Most of us do not live a life of monastic rigor, our days are full of jagged edges and jangling moments. But in some way we all have little rituals that shape our day—how we move through the morning, end the evening, etc. We do not often value what we may call 'routines' as rituals—to us they are too ordinary. Far from honoring them, we pay them no heed. We see them only as routines, not as paths to awareness."[37]

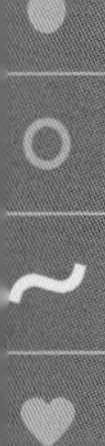

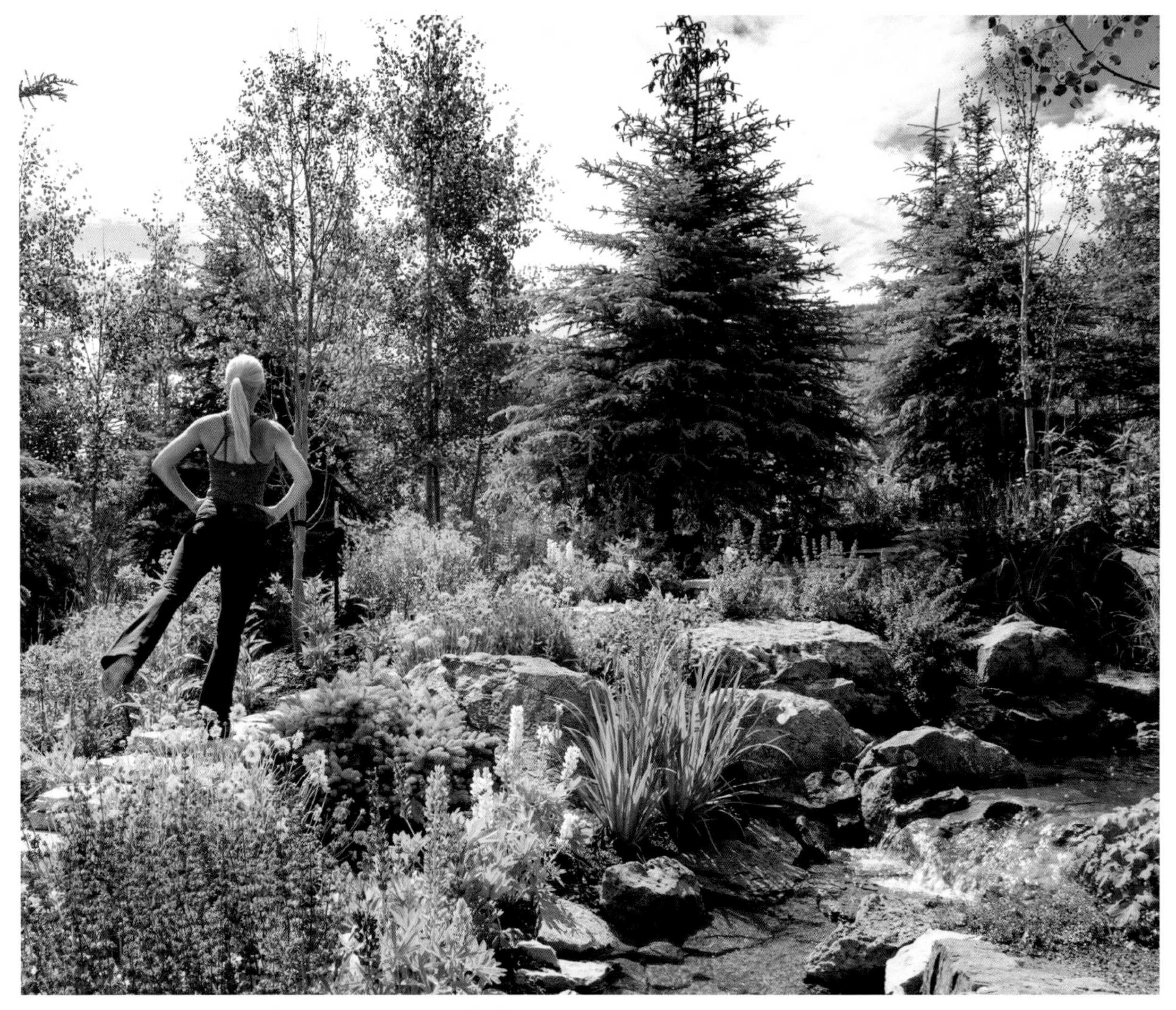

Sometimes you must go on faith, trusting that your body may know more than you do, trusting that the future holds better things than you thought may be possible.

2. **Suspend your thoughts.** How do you stop your clever mind from sabotaging you, with the gazillion creative reasons you should not work out today? You *just do it*.
   - With a schedule set for your workouts, tell yourself there is no reason to revisit it. It's time to show up—for you and for God—everyday.
   - Once you arrive to work out, know that your spirit will be lifted and you will have greater resolve than you could have predicted you would.
   - Our bodies are designed to enjoy muscle memory, in which tasks become easier over time as we start to remember movements at a cellular level. How miraculous is that? Live by faith. *Your body may know more than you do about what you can do!*
3. **Compartmentalize.** Don't allow drama to deter you from your goals and from the vision you have for yourself. Try not to allow a family argument, a work stress or a dilemma with which you are wrestling to color the determination you bring to your fitness. Whatever the problem may be, set it aside for a half-hour. You will be better able to manage it if you are healthy, calm and have added energy—all of which are side effects of daily exercise.

People have asked me for years, how do I *believe* that I can do the things I set out to do? Where does the confidence come from that enables me to overcome obstacles and remain on my path?

As I mentioned before, the longest distance I had ever run before the 26.2 marathon I completed was 16.5 miles. And when I climbed Mt. Kilimanjaro, I had three children at home under the age of eight. Though I did carry them on my back during some of my training, I assure you that I wasn't climbing mountains everyday with them, like something out of *The Sound of Music*—one of my favorite movies, by the way.

For me, every big dream begins with a plan of action—and breaking big ideas into small, manageable pieces, the way I just showed you how to do with your exercise. This is how I keep myself from getting overwhelmed: I put one foot in front of another. I show up, and let grace take over.

WALK OUT IN FAITH

Now it's your turn to let grace take over. When you take your walk around the neighborhood tonight, think about the power of *pause, think and act*. Of walking away, moving on and living your life on your own terms. Of finding the strength that dances within us, which can overcome so many obstacles we put in God's way. Know that when we suspend our thoughts, leave behind the perpetual buzz of computer screens and phones and walk instead by faith, we are filled.

Tomorrow, be the person who jumps out of bed in the morning, eager to find the sacred in everything around you. Use your body, and show up to experience fresh air, sunshine, laughter and sweat. Cultivate your fitness as a matter of faith. Move every day, appreciating what a profound gift each day *really is*.

Live for Others

A MESSAGE OF PURPOSE & COMMUNITY

"The divine sings in our good deeds."
—*Rabbi Abraham Heschel*

With the final pillar, we live for others. Indeed, researchers tell us, when we tend to our neighbor in the form of volunteer service, we also tend to ourselves. Not only is volunteering immensely powerful for the spirit, it has proven benefits for our physical bodies.

No gift is ever too small. No contribution is ever too insignificant to improve the quality of life for another. When I first entered the business world, I volunteered to lead the United Way campaign in the large company where I worked. John Mentzer, a gracious man who was retired and volunteering full time with the campaign, shared this story with me—"The Star Thrower," by Joel Barker. It has forever changed my life, and I still carry the account John gave me, now tattered, in my wallet—see the photo on the right. Here is my simplified version of this inspiring parable:

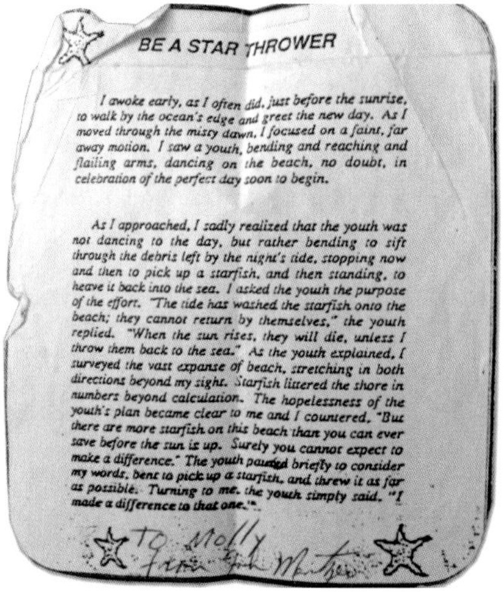

> A man who lived at the beach woke up early one foggy and drizzly morning. He looked out his window and could see a child dancing in the surf, off in the distance. He was captivated by the sight and decided to take a walk along the shore which was covered with starfish. As he got closer, he realized the child wasn't dancing at all but, instead, was throwing starfish into the ocean.
>
> He approached the girl and asked why he was doing such a thing. The child replied that it was low tide and if she didn't get the starfish back into the ocean, they were going to die. Perplexed, the man explained that there were thousands of starfish out that morning and that the girl couldn't possibly make a difference. She looked up at him, picked up a starfish, tossed it back into the sea and said, "I made a difference to that one."

BE A STAR THROWER

I awoke early, as I often did, just before the sunrise, to walk by the ocean's edge and greet the new day. As I moved through the misty dawn, I focused on a faint, far away motion. I saw a youth, bending and reaching and flailing arms, dancing on the beach, no doubt, in celebration of the perfect day soon to begin.

As I approached, I sadly realized that the youth was not dancing to the day, but rather bending to sift through the debris left by the night's tide, stopping now and then to pick up a starfish, and then standing, to heave it back into the sea. I asked the youth the purpose of the effort. "The tide has washed the starfish onto the beach; they cannot return by themselves," the youth replied. "When the sun rises, they will die, unless I throw them back to the sea." As the youth explained, I surveyed the vast expanse of beach, stretching in both directions beyond my sight. Starfish littered the shore in numbers beyond calculation. The hopelessness of the youth's plan became clear to me and I countered, "But there are more starfish on this beach than you can ever save before the sun is up. Surely you cannot expect to make a difference." The youth paused briefly to consider my words, bent to pick up a starfish, and threw it as far as possible. Turning to me, the youth simply said, "I made a difference to that one."

To Molly

YOU AND STARFISH TOSSING

If you are not yet plucking starfish off the beach and tossing them back into the living water, one by one, the world needs you to start.

Volunteering can have a profound, unseen and unexpected impact on your life and the lives of others. It's a way to share your talents, skills and abilities to help others, with no expectation of being paid.

Selfless in nature, volunteering nevertheless brings rich rewards. Leading a docent tour at a museum or mentoring an inner city child, you'll gain a better understanding of the world and expand your point of view. And that's just for starters!

THE PROVEN BENEFITS OF VOLUNTEERING

So far I've asked you to drink copious amounts of water, to eat the fruits and veggies of God's green earth and to exercise daily. As part of a 21-day plan to transform your body and increase your energy, these tenets make sense, right? But, you may wonder, how is it possible for your physiology to be altered by writing a card to a service member who is deployed overseas? How could your blood pressure be lowered by contributing a casserole to your church's monthly dinner at a domestic abuse shelter?

The connection between volunteering and good health may sound unconventional but there is growing evidence that it does, in fact, exist. Here's what scientific research shows:

Extend Your Life, Improve Your Overall Health. In a study of 1,000 adults, Carnegie Mellon University researchers found that volunteering regularly:

- Cut the risk of the adults' high blood pressure by 40 percent
- Lowered overall mortality risk by 47 percent
- Likely also lowered the risk of depression and anxiety
- Bolstered psychological well-being.

The type of volunteering did not matter, *but the hours you put in were important*. The Carnegie Mellon study identified the benefits in adults who volunteered 200 hours or more each year.

Volunteering helps you stay physically healthy. It's good for us at any age, but especially for older adults. Studies show that older adults do extend their lives by volunteering, even when considering factors like the health of the participants. Volunteering also decreases symptoms of chronic pain or heart disease.[38]

Canadian researchers recently found, in a study of more than 100 teens, that volunteering over a 10-week period led to a drop in cholesterol, body mass index and inflammation. "The volunteers who reported the greatest increases in empathy, altruistic behavior and mental health were the ones who also saw the greatest improvements in their cardiovascular health," Hannah Schreier, Ph.D., said.[39]

Some of these benefits are from staying physically and mentally active, but serving others is also a social, purpose-driven activity—which likely releases our feel-good hormones such as oxytocin and lowers those pesky stress hormones, such as cortisol.[40] Yes, low cortisol, the condition that often leads to binge eating and wild calorie sprees.

Get Happy. The more you volunteer, the happier you get. That's what researchers at the London School of

Economics found when they studied the relationship between service work and measures of happiness in a large group of American adults. Compared with people who didn't volunteer, the odds of being "very happy" rose 7 percent among those who volunteered monthly and 12 percent for people who volunteered every two to four weeks. Among weekly volunteers, 16 percent felt very happy—a hike in happiness comparable to having an income of $75,000-$100,000 versus $20,000, say the researchers. Devoting time to religious organizations had the greatest impact.[41]

It's a poignant paradox. If we make less money than we would prefer to make, but we go out and work for others for free, our life satisfaction lifts so much that it feels as though we are wealthier. That sounds like one of those twist-and-turn parables that Jesus is always using to illustrate his points. *Exactly.*

Serving is what I believe *we were built to do*. As we become more closely aligned to the purpose God intends for our lives, we can enhance our health, extend our lives and markedly improve our happiness. The less we make life about us, the more we encounter the divine. The more disciplined we become about living for our neighbor, the more transcendent our lives become.

I'm sure this seems quirky to you—the idea that you turned to me and this book for weight loss and fitness advice and you've encountered a ministry of sorts. Yet, this is the unconventional truth, more and more of which science is revealing to us. We are at our best, physically and spiritually, when we devote more of our lives to saving the world, one starfish at a time.

THE COMBINED POWER OF THE PILLARS

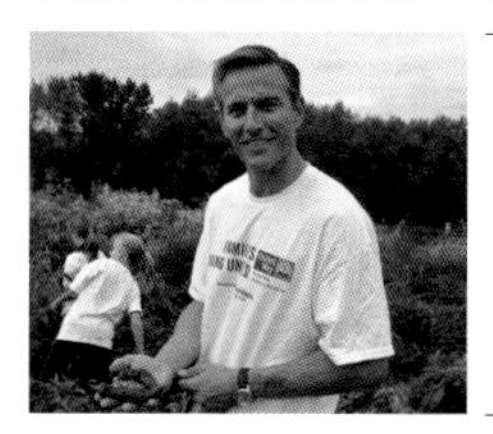

Dean
AGE 47
OCCUPATION Real Estate Company President
HOMETOWN Annapolis, MD

Dean is a 47-year-old president of a real estate company in Maryland. He was already a fan of working out and spending time at the gym before he attended a Molly Vibrant Living workshop. Dean liked the idea of becoming more intentional about his health, and added the pillars into his life one at a time. "The water piece was intriguing to me, the way that Molly said it would impact everything with my health."

Within a short time, Dean started losing weight and he felt considerably better. He stopped getting headaches he had often experienced before, simply from drinking much more water. So he added in the second pillar—eating REAL. Within a few months, Dean lost 25 pounds, weight he has now kept off for more than a year. "For me, the pillars of the program seemed to build on themselves. To eat real, I started cooking."

Dean was going through a divorce at the time—and had not previously done much cooking. He was literally starting from scratch, learning how to make meals instead of relying on take-out for himself, his 17-year-old daughter and his 12-year-old son. "The prep of a meal became more of an event at our house," Dean says. "I came to cherish those times, getting involved in making dinner with the kids."

For Dean, the fourth pillar came very easily, as he was already involved in the community. But he got much

GET STARTED LIVING FOR OTHERS

If planned charitable activities in your community don't fit your schedule, take the lead and find ways to help local shelters, food pantries or schools. Not only can you gain personal satisfaction from giving of yourself, you set an example for others to follow.

Identify something you care about and find a way to make a difference. If you like reading, teach someone to read. If you like cooking, set a quarterly date with friends or colleagues to make healthy casseroles and personally deliver them to families in need.

More Volunteer Suggestions:

- Donate blood through your local American Red Cross.
- Mentor a child through Big Brothers or Big Sisters.
- Be an active role model for a colleague at work who could use your support.
- Write letters to members of the military stationed overseas.
- Host a healthy food drive and donate items to local food pantries and schools.
- Volunteer at your local animal shelter.
- Bake cookies and hand deliver them to residents at an elderly care facility.
- Contact your local United Way for volunteer opportunities.
- Give of your time at a local farm.
- Go to volunteermatch.org and enter your zip code as well as areas of interest to be matched with an organization seeking your help.
- Specific, work-related talents like accounting, web design, and Microsoft Excel® are also needed at many non-profit organizations. Go to catchafire.org to find out where you can be of service.

more active in volunteering, incorporating his new appreciation for healthy eating. Charged with bringing brown rice to a Stone Soup event, the details of which I will soon share, Dean didn't have a big pot. "I think I spent four or five hours making rice that first time. Then I got a bigger rice pot!"

I cherish the image of this devoted man, hovering over small pans or rice much of the day, all so that he could bring his promised component for the greater good. He was tossing starfish and the task became absorbing!

Switching it up—from a small to a big rice pot—worked for Dean. But how will you structure your life—likely already bulging with obligations—so that you can add not one, not two, not three, but *four* pillars, the last one of which is a hearty amount of volunteer service? As you have seen, I love structure. I love planning,

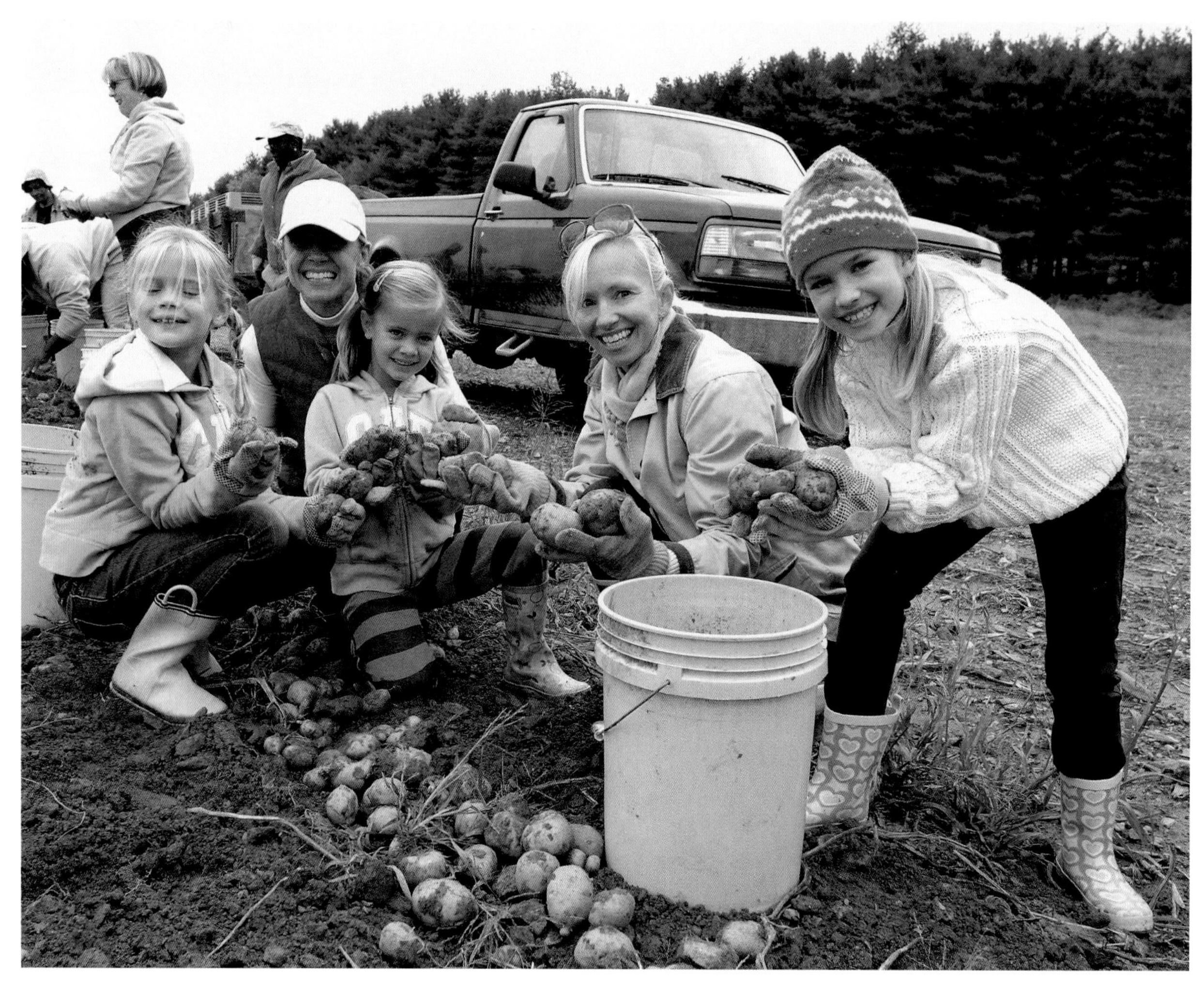

Lillian and I (on right) with close friends, Casey, Lindy and Emily, gleaning potatoes. Volunteering reorients your life so that it's not all about you. If it gets you outside, burning calories and focusing on healthier lifestyle choices, it's a win-win.

compartmentalizing and slotting healthy habits into my life so that I don't have to think about health and fitness, because it is carried forward in my schedule and embedded in my lifestyle.

STRUCTURING YOUR SERVICE

It's been nearly nine years since I have had a child in diapers, yet I still carry a diaper bag as a handbag. That's how much I crave structure in my life—all those little cubbies, into which I can tuck my water bottle, my baggies of nuts, my lip gloss and a host of other easy-to-find items. Fortunately, there are a host of fabulous chic diaper bags on the market today so I don't have to sacrifice style in my quest for ultimate domination of the sundry stuff in my life. That's just how I roll.

I want *you* to have more structure in your life—healthy scaffolding which the 21-Day Action Plan can help you build and sustain. When it comes to living for others, here's the structured steps I recommend.

1. Pick service projects that play to your passion. Research shows that when you serve as a volunteer, you will reap the biggest health benefits if your work is in-line with your most cherished beliefs. That's why, scientists think, faith-based volunteerism seems to be a particularly potent healer. *Your circuitry responds when your work is electrified by your passion.*

When I work with clients in the 21-Day Action Plan, I invite them to join me at a variety of community service projects I'm involved in. That way, they have a familiar face or two on which to rely, as they embark on projects they know little about, and as they enter communities and neighborhoods they don't usually encounter.

One of my passions is food. I like to spend much of my volunteer time feeding, not just homeless citizens, but also the enormous number of people in our communities who cannot count on having three nutritious meals each day. This is called food insecurity. In essence, many of our neighbors, people in houses and apartments just like you and me, run low on funds each month and cannot always afford groceries, especially those foods that are healthy.

The more we expose ourselves to these ideas—that real food is precious, that the earth and its bounty are utterly linked to our health, and that we all eat from this common source—the more we will change ourselves, the planet and our communities in need.

The Spiritual Discipline of Gleaning

In Biblical times, the ritual of apportioning some of your harvest to the widows, orphans and the less fortunate, was called *gleaning*:

"Now when you reap the harvest of your land, you shall not reap to the very corners of your field, nor shall you gather the gleanings of your harvest. Nor shall you glean your vineyard, nor shall you gather the fallen fruit of your vineyard; you shall leave them for the needy and for the stranger. I am the Lord your God." (Leviticus 19: 9-10)

As you have seen in the previous pillars, reviving our agricultural roots—and the appreciation that we are from the land and that everything we need comes from the earth—has enormous implications for the way we live our lives. I believe that the most vulnerable members of our society need the most nutrient-rich, enlivening and enticing food we have to offer. If you need health and energy to improve your life circumstances, a diet of processed food is not much help. So as tempting as it is to give to a food bank the discards from our pantries—the canned goods we bought on impulse and didn't like, or the rejects we no longer want to include in our diets—I've devoted a significant amount of my community service work to a higher standard of food for those in need.

In Baltimore, I help promote and organize gleaning events, in which urban and suburban dwellers, moms and scout troops, corporations and families spend a few hours on farms inside and outside the city harvesting bushels of fruits and vegetables leftover after the choice produce has been professionally culled from the fields and the orchards. I love these *days of caring*—getting exercise doing physical work, sinking my hands into the soil, being outdoors and gathering these jewels from the earth for the nourishment of others' bodies.

Stone Soup

One of the other events I started in my community is called Stone Soup, based on the book which calls on each household in a village to bring a single ingredient and out of which the villagers create a hearty soup that feeds all of them.

The best part of Stone Soup is counting all the meals we prepare—shouting out to the assembled, "We made 278 lentil casseroles! 220 chicken and broccoli dishes! 1,259 veggie snack bags!" It is a loaves and fishes moment, the divine channeled through us in a flourish of beautiful food.

After these events, we are ready to celebrate. When we have done what God intends, and filled our day with care for God's children, then it's time to share a joyful meal together with family and friends, basking in the memories of the day.

Passion-Fueled Life Lessons

The life lessons these two service projects engender are enormous. With gleaning, we see that throughout history, communities took it upon themselves to identify waste and to make nourishment possible for those in need. And you get connected to the farm, the earth and the source of your strength and sustenance. With Stone Soup, volunteers are asked to bring healthy ingredients—whole grain rice instead of white rice, cut-up fresh carrots and red peppers instead of potato chips, etc.—and to make dishes from scratch, rather than opening boxes of Rice-a-Roni™ or other prepared mixes. In this way, we educate the volunteer at the same time as we introduce better nutrition into the shelters and soup kitchens.

Whether it is gleaning, soup, picking up trash in a park or petitioning people to rid your community of a pervasive problem, your body and your spirit will best be served by your attending to your passions. So take some time to consider this today: What truly moves you, heart and soul? What work could you do in your life that you would consider the greatest privilege on earth?

2. Create a virtuous circle. To successfully structure any change in life, you need a circle of support. It could be that you invite some girlfriends over to your house to start cooking with real food. It could be that you

SPREAD THE LOVE

Here are two worthwhile volunteer activities that you could help organize in your community.

Stone Soup Event

In the "Stone Soup" children's story, hungry soldiers enter a village in search of a dry place to sleep. After being told by all the villagers there was no food to eat or place to lay their heads, they put a pot of water on a fire to boil and put a big stone in the pot. The villagers grew curious and one by one, they began contributing ingredients until they had assembled a hearty meal for all of the community to feast on.

Nearly four years ago, this book's theme inspired my kids and I to create Stone Soup as an event for Families Living United in Maryland, and the movement has grown to being promoted world-wide through the United Way. With the same idea as the book, we ask 150 volunteers to contribute ingredients for our healthy recipes (casseroles, harvest mix, veggie snack bags, etc.) and to join us in making the food at a local shelter for the hungry families in our community. The 2-hour event takes place at a local shelter, and we've found it creates an immediate sense of community connection for volunteers of all ages. The activity then sparks a long-term interest among the volunteers, expanding the impact we can have on our neighbors in need.

For more information about hosting a Stone Soup event, check out all the logistics on my website at www.mollyshattuck.com.

Healthy Food Drives

Spring and summer months are an extremely slow time for food donations, leaving shelters, food banks/pantries and soup kitchens with empty shelves. But the need for healthy food is growing at an alarming rate across our nation. In central Maryland alone, more than 325,000 children and adults do not have adequate nutrition or access to healthy foods. Together with the United Way of Central Maryland, we offer the Access to Healthy Food Initiative to increase the sourcing and distribution of healthy food for people who need it. One of the ways we do this is by hosting healthy food drives. Get all the details so you, too, can set up a food drive in your community. Find them at www.mollyshattuck.com.

I always love to learn new ways to be of service and help those in my community. Let us know about one of your most rewarding volunteer experiences by discussing it in the **Vibrant Living Community** at www.mollyshattuck.com.

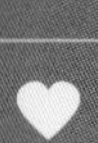

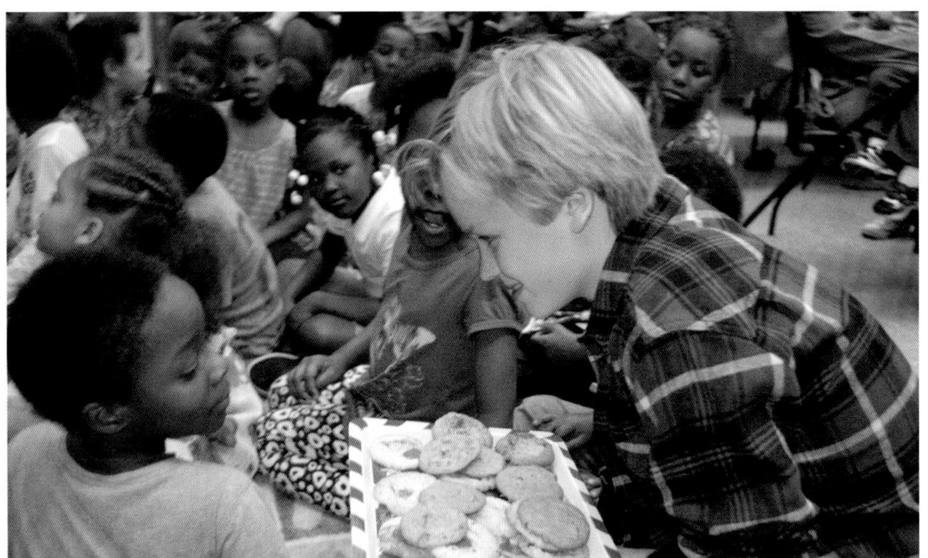

My son, Wyatt, serving cookies and my daughter, Lillian, reading to children at a local shelter. Choose to live *your* life in gratitude. We are all in this world together, and we need one another.

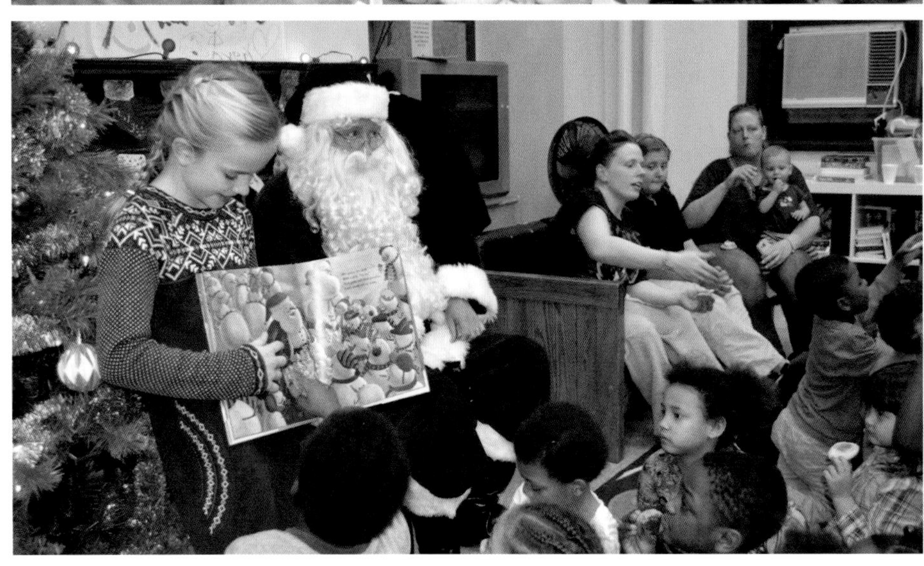

identify some work mates who would be willing to walk with you at lunch, or hold you accountable for your after-hours workouts. Telling people in your life about your goals and inviting supportive—not toxic—friends to be "on your team" will propel you to success with all four pillars.

I cultivate connections with people like this in my life, and I call them my *virtuous circle*. In fact, I rely on several virtuous circles every day—the circle of my family; the circle of some lifelong, longstanding friends; the circle of volunteers I serve alongside; and the circle of exercise buddies and clients I work out with, among others. Friends who want to see you healthy won't balk at being asked to walk with you in the park, instead of going out to eat or watching TV at home. Friends who truly "get" you will go along with you on volunteer service. They will eagerly refill your water bottle before you get on the road for your traffic-snarled drive home. The little ways we care for one another are paid forward so that the circle grows bigger and bigger, the impact on our communities more and more expansive.

For me, the energy of a virtuous circle is utterly intoxicating. It is an incomparable kind of energy—the circle of community and caring we create together. That is what I so often feel when I volunteer. Let me tell you a rather long story, but one that best conveys the torrent of energy a virtuous circle can create.

The Power of Love

In 2006, my second year of cheering for the NFL, the Baltimore Ravens organization sponsored and volunteered for Habitat for Humanity, gutting and restoring a four-bedroom house in East Baltimore. The cheerleaders, players and the front office staff signed up for three-hour stints each week for seven weeks, hammering wallboard into place, painting windowsills and contributing other physical labor.

One day when I was leaving, a man and his daughter arrived and shared with me that the place we were renovating was going to be their house. They were part of a family that had been displaced by Hurricane Katrina and had since been shuttled from shelter to shelter and in and out of temporary housing in horrific experiences they went on to describe. The man's wife, too, had recently been diagnosed with breast cancer and was undergoing chemotherapy in Baltimore, where they had been resettled into a church-sponsored shelter. Now after their year-long ordeal, Habitat for Humanity had picked them to receive a home and they were ecstatic.

Habitat was supplying a four-bedroom house for this family of seven, the husband, wife and their four children—one of whom had a baby herself. But the home would come unfurnished and this family had nothing, in essence having been refugees for more than a year, carrying what they had from shelter to shelter.

Pause. Think. Act.

Before Ty Pennington and the "Extreme Makeover Home Edition" team had skyrocketed, I had a crazy vision: *What if we surprised this family with a completely furnished, utterly stocked home?*

I went to cheer practice that night and started rallying the troops. I penned an email to the entire Ravens organization, local companies and friends with a comprehensive list of everything we would need for the home. Immediately, the email responses to help came flooding in.

Originally from Louisiana, free safety Ed Reed responded in a big way to people in need from his home state: "What size are the beds? I'll go buy the mattresses."

Steve and Renee Bisciotti, the owners of the Ravens, paid for the appliances—the washer, dryer, and the oven. Tony Pashos, then an offensive lineman with the Ravens, pledged to move furniture, hang blinds—whatever was needed.

I wish I had room to acknowledge the avalanche of donations that arrived, many large contributions from Constellation Energy employees, from well-heeled and imposing NFL players but also from an ever-expanding crowd of people who jumped in to offer embroidered tea towels and a host of other small and thoughtful gifts. All of it got dropped off in my garage where my three children—the oldest of which was 7 at that time—inventoried everything with clipboards, Wyatt wearing his treasured Bob the Builder hard hat.

The Big Reveal

We had only one day to set up, between the time the house was finished and the time the family was scheduled to move in. Every new cabinet had to be scoured and then stocked—with all the groceries Safeway donated. The coffeemaker, toaster, hand mixer, tea towels, plates, silverware, pots and pans were set lovingly inside. The donated mattresses were made up with colorful new sheets and comforters; the girls' rooms were decorated with bright curtains, donated art and chic lamps. A bassinet, changing table, diapers and pacifiers were put into place. I made a wreath to hang on the front door. And the biggest teddy bear in the NFL, Tony Pashos, walked out of the kitchen, carrying warm homemade chocolate-chip cookies we had baked for the family to coincide with their arrival.

To see the teenage daughters tear through that home, squealing with happiness, as mom and dad wept with joy, was a moment so exhilarating, I felt weightless. The pinnacle moment? When all seven of them jumped in glee on the mom and dad's bed, shouting, "We're finally home!"

Talk about energy! It remains one of the single happiest moments of my life, right up there with seeing my babies born and reaching the summit of Kilimanjaro, the fourth tallest mountain in the world. Let me tell you, I've been exposed to some incredible energy before. There were times, cheering before 70,000 screaming NFL football fans—mind you, in white go-go boots and a skirt that's only nine inches long—I felt I could literally be transported yards across the stadium by the roar of the crowd alone.

> Yet for me, there's no bigger adrenaline rush than that of living for others and filling your time with good deeds.

And remarkably, the good deed—the *mitzvah*, as Jewish friends call it—heals the giver as much as it does the recipient. Because as it turns out, I lost six pounds in a mere two weeks, so much so that the Ravens cheerleading coach called me in to inquire about my weight loss and to warn me to lose no more or I wouldn't be cheering at the next game.

It is so very true that many hands make light work. Living for others, for perfect strangers and people who you may never meet or know, is a feather-light task when you are part of a circle of people who want to pay it forward. Ask yourself right now:

- Who in my life offers an unconditional source of support?
- Who will be my cheerleader?
- If you don't have enough of those people in your life, where might you turn to expand your virtuous circle?
- Who might volunteer with me and expand my circle?

3. Build higher purpose into whatever you do. You may be juggling a lot of plates right now—and it may not be realistic, financially sound or family-friendly for you to devote a great deal of time to volunteering. But whatever you spend every day of your life doing, infuse it with a commitment to something bigger than yourself.

So you want to drink more water. Let's say that you set a goal for yourself—you're going to drink 80 ounces of water every day and you calculate that in a month, you will consume 2,400 ounces of water and in five months nearly 10,000 ounces. What if you established that each time you reach an interval of 10,000 ounces, you will make a micro-loan to support a water-purification or transport project somewhere in the world? On www.kiva.org, you can lend $25 and support individuals around the globe who are creating livelihoods for their families with your help. When you set your sights on something bigger than yourself, your personal goals become decidedly more meaningful and a lot more fun.

Change Your Purpose, Change Your Point of View

In the same way that water and veggies displace soda and fries, selfless service draws us away from the mall, the mirror and, ultimately, from self-absorption. In our society, we have so many temptations to over-consume, to over-buy and to become dazzled by the importance of "things," drama and other pretenses.

> With volunteer work, I have found, we are drawn to higher purpose living, to the precious task of nurturing growth and health in others.

The author Bradley Wigger writes, "Personally, I believe acts of service teach the deepest lessons in the mystery of others and consequently are one of the greatest weapons against evil." Indeed, there are so many lessons to be gleaned from service.

Finding ways to connect yourself with the greater good sets into motion a fundamental behavior change. If, for example, emotional eating has sabotaged your weight loss efforts in the past, a volunteer engagement can take your mind off whatever worries might besiege you when you are at home and in close proximity to the fridge. If lack of follow-through with exercise has proved your downfall, seeing the struggles of others or the constancy of a long-time volunteer may inspire you to dig deeper within yourself for resolve.

Set Your Purpose High

Over the years, as I have shared, I have set a number of goals for myself. In some cases, I tied the goal to a higher purpose—something bigger than me and the accomplishment at hand. When I ran my first marathon, for example, I raised money for the Leukemia Society, a cause near and dear to me, having had friends with leukemia.

Similarly, when I climbed Mt. Kilimanjaro, I wanted the cause to be more as meaningful as the climb. As I began to research it, there were all sorts of expeditions and groups I could join. But nothing proved more compelling than the Climate Change Expedition—a mission to bring weather-monitoring equipment to the highest point in Africa to study the effects of global warming.

I arrived in Tanzania and met, for the first time, the nine companions with whom I would be climbing for the next six or seven days. As you can imagine, we were a cast of characters, and my fellow climbers razzed me plenty for applying lip gloss and wearing color-coordinated outfits—even my hats matched—on our ascent. Over the course of the week, we grew very close as you inevitably do when you are climbing all day, sleeping, cooking, pooping and peeing together in the great outdoors. So when my fellow climber Paul developed too much knee pain to continue the climb, he asked me to take the ashes of a loved one (which a good friend of his entrusted him to spread at the top of the mountain.)

It was an exhilarating week, and one I had dreamed about since I first read Ernest Hemingway's "Snows of Kilimanjaro" in high school. I was carrying with me a letter from my children and stuffed bears they sent with me for good luck. In my pack were a few little shreds of pom poms the cheerleaders had collected from the Ravens' practice facility and sent with me on my journey to Africa. Buoyed by the prayers and good wishes of so many friends, and of the scientific community, we installed and flicked on the switch of the weather tracking equipment for the first time nearly 15,000 feet above sea level. And at the summit, overlooking craters and glaciers as far as the eye could see and hearing the eerie sound of glaciers shifting and melting, I spread Paul's friend's ashes. In my quest to make a trip of deep meaning and purpose, I found there was room for even more sacred souvenirs.

DWELLING TOGETHER ON THIS GREEN EARTH

You can wedge into your life pockets of beauty and intense gratification. Volunteering and seeking out opportunities to be God's hands in the world will expose you to untold benefits—to your mood, to your outlook and to your health. When you devote your life to others, you will feel the divine coursing through you, and it will transform you.

Thich Nhat Hanh, the Buddhist monk, said, "The miracle is not that Jesus walked on water. The miracle is that Jesus walked *on the green earth* . . . The miracle is *dwelling deeply in the present moment and feeling truly alive*." We, too, have the miracle of walking this green earth—of being truly alive and dwelling with others. We can harvest food and break bread together. We can create a virtuous circle, moving together and making peace, as God intended us to do.

"Remember that when you leave this earth, you take with you nothing that you have received—only what you have given."

—*Francis of Assisi*

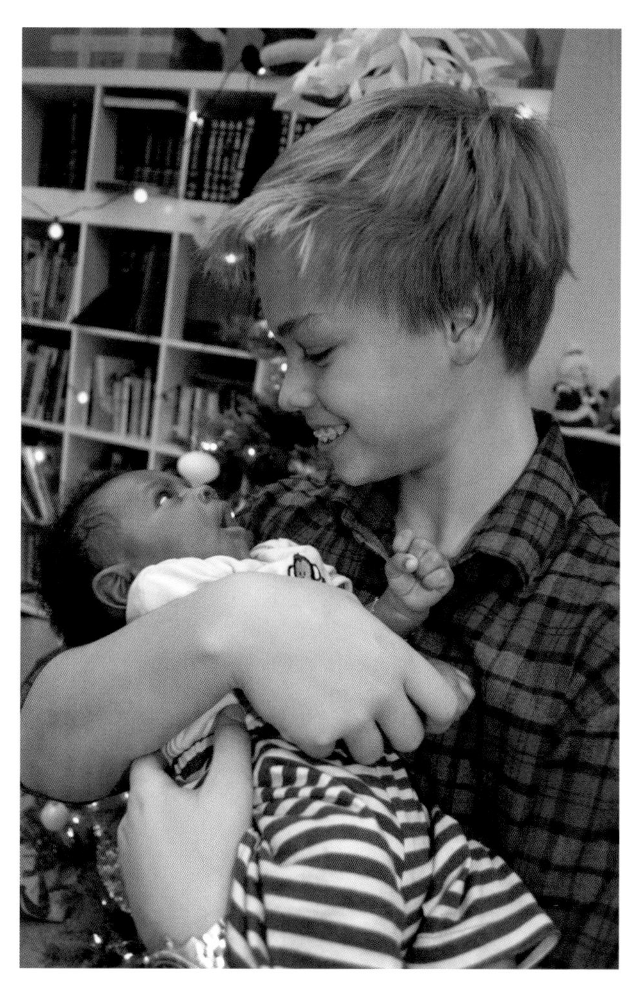

My oldest boy Spencer and a sweet baby at one of our shelter parties. We can learn so much from children who, seemingly from birth, are naturally imbued with a love of others, regardless of differences or circumstances.

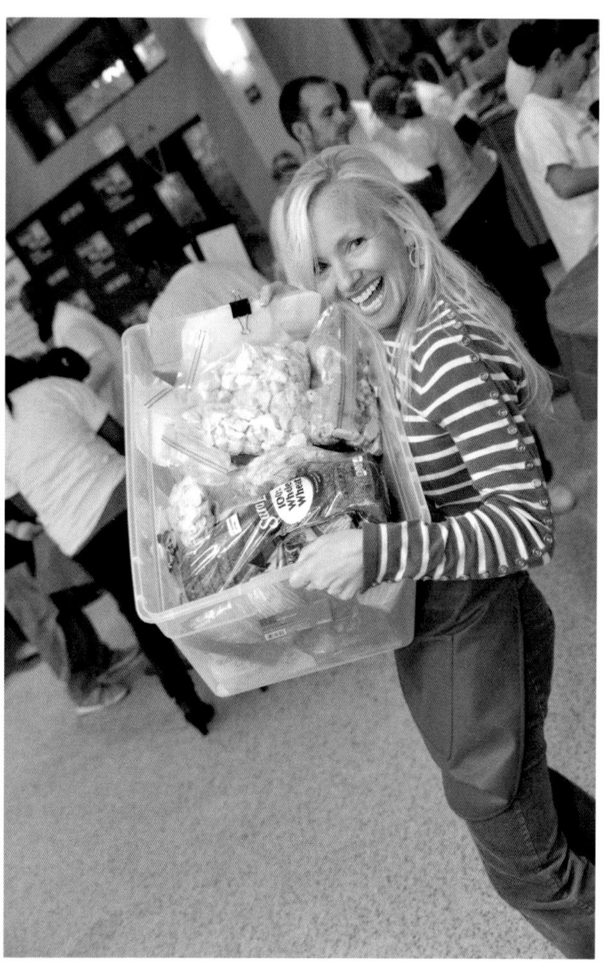

Me at one of our Stone Soup events at Our Daily Bread—a magnificent organizations in Baltimore committed to improving the lives of people in need.

Four Pillars and the Virtuous Circle

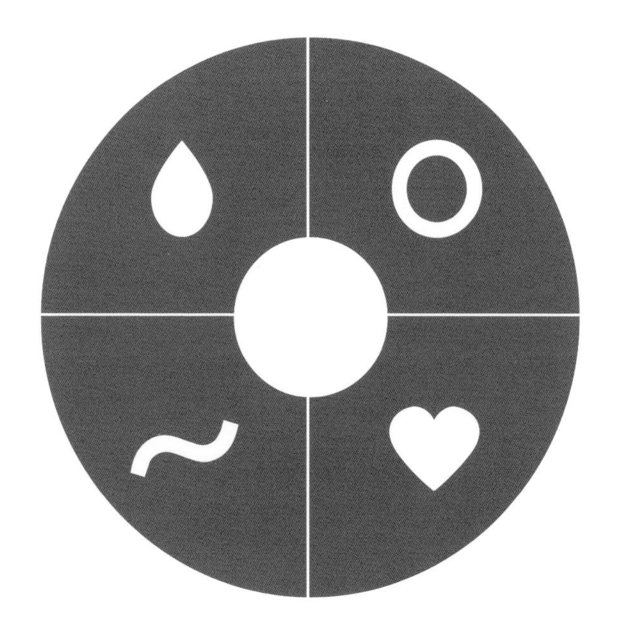

"We have the best discussions at school," my 14-year-old son Spencer remarked recently. I love that thought-provoking talks have a "cool factor" for my teen. But I also believe there's a hidden dynamic in his classrooms, promoting free dialogue. What is it? The students and teachers at Spencer's school sit around a large circular table—it's called the Harkness method of teaching—rather than the typical set-up in which the teacher stands in front of the students.

What is it about a circle that is so powerful? In a circle, we act in mutual respect and in balanced proportion. Fittingly, the circle shape abounds in nature. The earth, moon, planets and stars. Tangerines and tomatoes. Peas and blueberries. Water droplets and bubbles. And of course, the circle of life.

Richly connected to the earth, circles are deeply spiritual, too. In grand cathedrals, the round, rose-adorned, stained glass windows evoke for us a sense of boundless love. In Native American dream catchers or in the Buddhist mandala, a circle seems to invite the opening of the soul and the setting aside of fear.

ELEMENTS IN BALANCE

The Molly Vibrant Living program relies on a *virtuous circle*. When we live in respect and balance with others, with the earth and with God, a very powerful synthesis occurs. I'm sure you've felt this power, too, in the love of a family circle, a group of girlfriends, or in a project that hums with synergy.

In our very core, I believe we all want to be connected to something bigger than ourselves. Regardless of how much we enjoy our solitude, we also thrive in community.

If it's too hard for us to name a new goal for ourselves, or if we don't have a group of go-to people in our lives, everything feels out of whack. Indeed, we feel left out of the circle, as if happiness, health, and opportunity are things that happen to *other* people.

YOU CREATE THE CIRCLE

But in reality, a virtuous circle is something *you* create, calling on the gifts God has given you. When you surround yourself with people who love and bring out the best in you, or when you fill your life with quality ingredients, you are more likely to feel what athletes describe as being "in the flow." Or what Zen Buddhists might call "being at one with things."

It is the same way with our bodies. We can cultivate a virtuous circle of habits that feed our energy, or we can choose to sap our strength with poor choices.

A virtuous circle of health is comprised of the four pillars we have just explored and which you will now be putting into practice: *water, real food, exercise and living for others.*

As you have seen, each of these pillars relates to and overlaps with the next. Indeed, these behaviors form a pattern that becomes chemical, neuron-writing and muscle-memory building. Infused with your gratitude for God's gifts in your life, the practice of the four pillars can also become a spiritual discipline, a way of acknowledging that you were built to love and serve.

In the next 21 days, you will get a glimpse of how these four main elements can change you physiologically. During this time, entertain the possibility that a balance built on these pillars might also attune you to greater life meaning and joy. Allow them to work in tandem, creating a circle of virtue and strength in the days to come.

Commit to be Faithfully Fit

Want to devote yourself to the pillars of healthy living? Here's 10 sure ways to do it.

1 Control your time.

Every person has the same amount of time in each day, week and year. How you choose to spend it makes all the difference. You have enough time for anything as long as it ranks high enough in your priorities. It's impossible to save time and quite easy to waste time, so get control!

2 Decide who is on your squad.

Surround yourself with a virtuous circle—positive people who support and cheer you on. Avoid those who have a negative attitude and rain down on your sunshine. Do not allow the people in your life to deplete your energy.

3 Forget about sit-ups.

Push-ups are the way to go! If done correctly (See the instructions on page 92), push-ups will turn a flabby tummy into a firm one. I had a hernia and haven't done a single sit-up since before I had children. Having gained 50 pounds with each pregnancy and enduring three cesarean sections, I found that push-ups were the key to getting my tummy toned.

4 You can do anything if you compartmentalize and focus.

Life and complicated projects can be overwhelming. Minimize the intimidation by setting mini goals and tackling them in smaller chunks. That way, you will experience continuous forward movement and higher productivity. All *big* goals start with baby steps. You must plan, organize, schedule, and be consistent—and don't stop until you reach your goal.

5 Make sleep a priority.

The quantity and quality of sleep we get has a direct impact on our mood, stress levels, and nutritional choices. Well-rested individuals are often happier, less stressed, and eat more healthfully. Prepare for a sound night's sleep by taking a relaxing bath or shower, free of the distractions of technology and dimly lit with candles or low light.

6 Tune out excessive info.

I rarely Google people (I would rather get to know them in person) or spend excessive time on-line, looking up information that doesn't matter. Keep your life real and don't get absorbed in time-consuming, mindless info-binging.

7 Touch it once.

Whatever it is that creates clutter in your life—mail, email, laundry, etc.—limit the number of steps involved. Pay the bills and answer the emails when they arrive. Avoid creating daunting piles of things that never get done. You may find you actually have the time to exercise because of how efficient you will become.

8 Smile and laugh every day.

You just might change someone's day (or life!) with a reassuring smile, and laughter increases the "feel good" hormones (endorphins and dopamine). At times, humor can help us cope with difficult situations and reduce stress, so laugh often!

9 Control what you can and have faith in every situation.

Life sometimes hits us hard, but don't allow a difficulty to define you or have an unlimited, energy-deflating lifespan. Make the most of every circumstance by finding the good and building on it. Don't ask God for an easier life. Ask God to make you a stronger person.

10 Find your passion and your purpose.

Giving selflessly can help you find and define your passion and mission in life. Allow yourself to be led into a higher-purpose life.

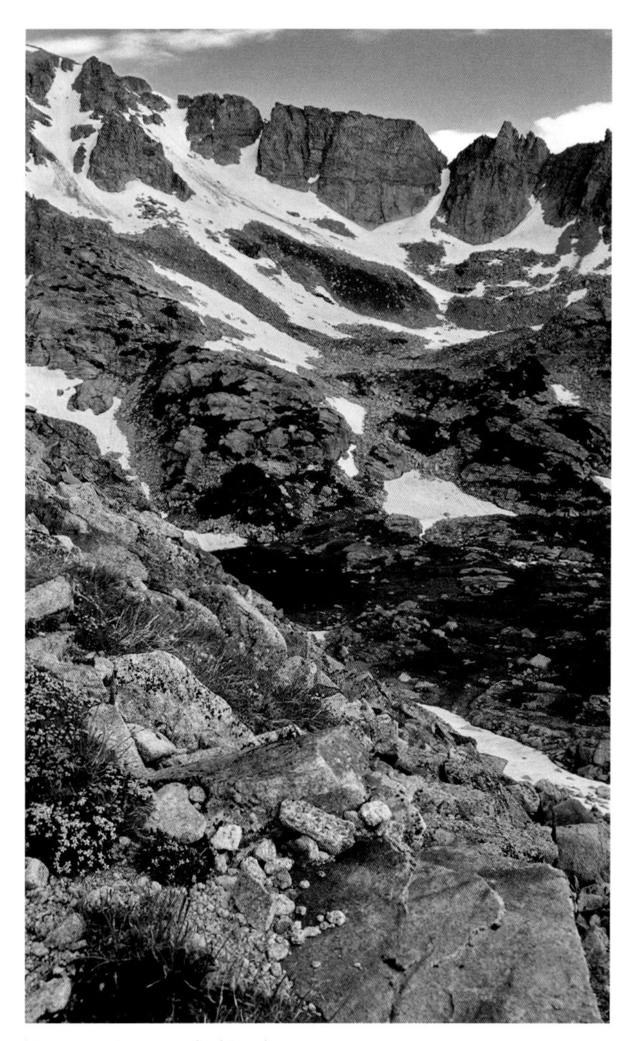

Lisa, my sister, took this photo in Colorado during a hike last summer.

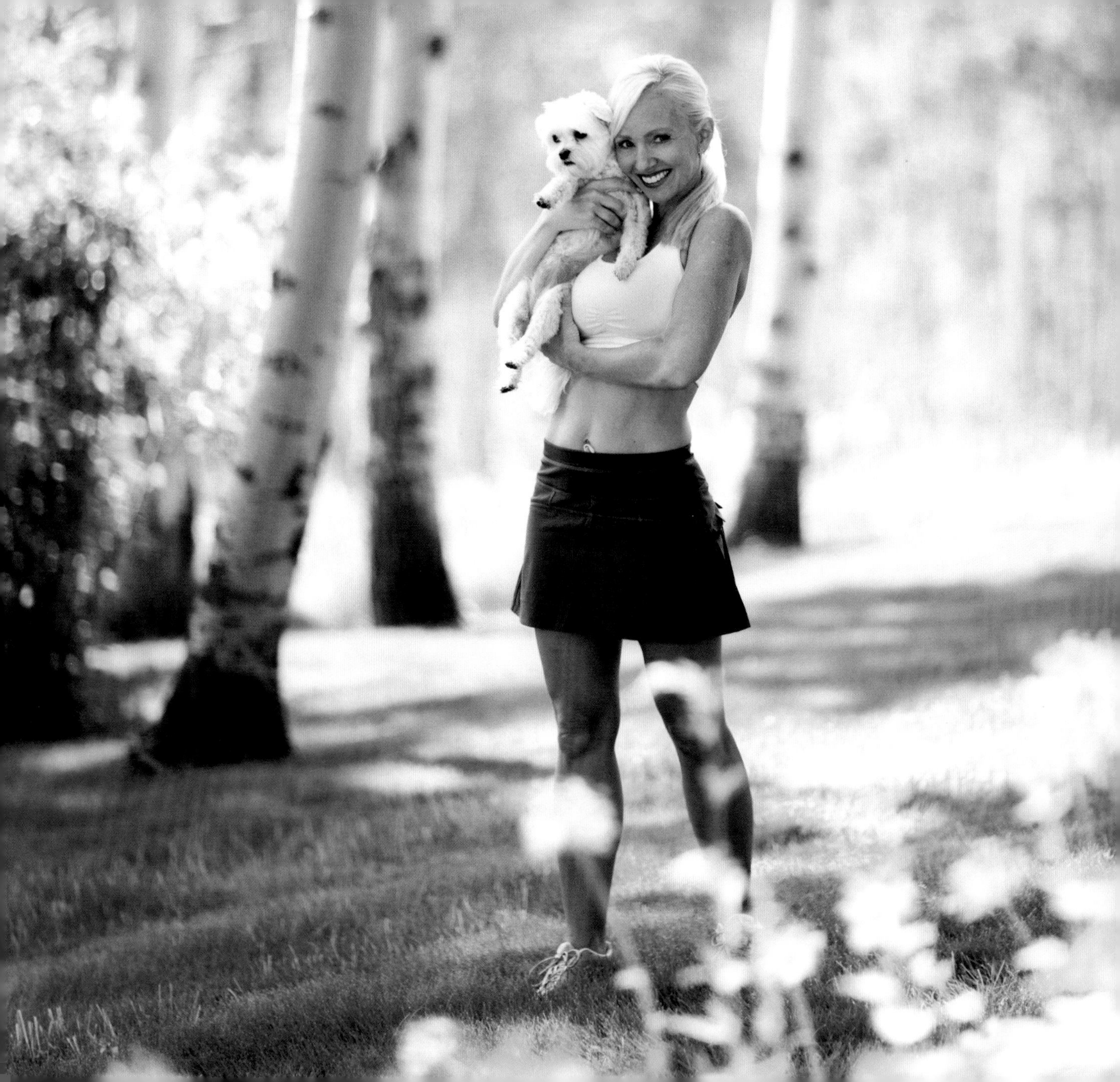

21-DAY ACTION PLAN

Get all the tools you need to launch your new habits: set your sights, stock your pantry, and gear up for great results.

Your Personal Goals

Personal health goals motivate us to be our best selves. And when we have a bad day—opting to devour a bag of chips instead of a juicy orange, or to plant your tush in a chair for hours on end and not get up to exercise—goals can help us get back on track.

You've decided to dedicate 21 days to creating healthy habits. Make the most of this opportunity by pushing yourself a little each day and being precise about the goals you want to achieve. On the next page you'll find a questionnaire to get you thinking about your health habits. Follow that up with your big goals for 21-Day Action Plan.

Take some time to decide what you want to accomplish and *write it down*. You need to be able to measure your progress, both short-term and long. So it's a good idea to set weekly mini goals and review your baby steps of progress.

Be realistic about what you can commit to doing. If, for example, you know it will be difficult to fit in the minimum 30 minutes of exercise I recommend, plan for the 20 minutes you know will work for you. You'll get the results you desire if you set realistic but challenging goals, follow the tips and recommendations in this book and make your goals a priority.

Planning, planning, planning — *no more excuses!*

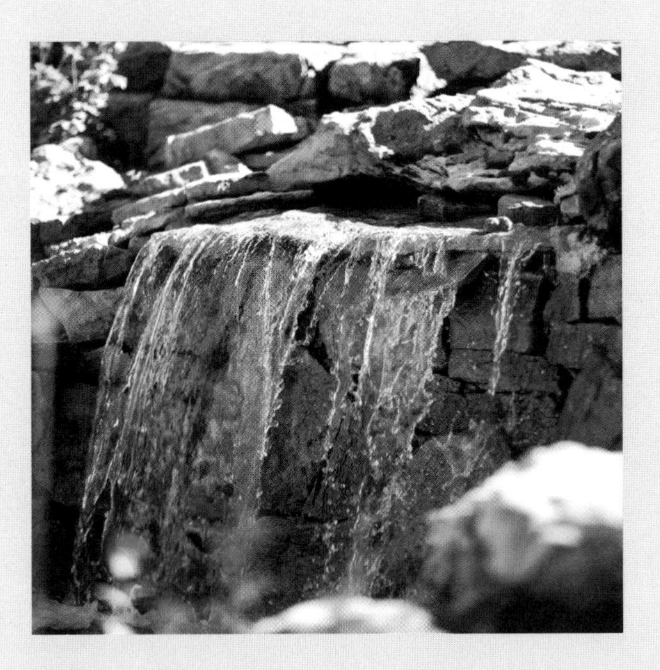

Simply outline your goals by writing them in the space provided below and commit to doing whatever it takes to become a healthier, stronger and more energized version of yourself.

No fibbing when you answer the questions below. This is for your eyes only, after all. That tape measure will eventually be your friend, even if the numbers are not yet in your favor. It's just a starting point!

QUESTIONNAIRE

Today's Date:

WEIGHT LOSS

What is your height?

How much do you weigh?

Do you want to lose weight during this 21-Day Action Plan? If so, how much?

What is your long-term goal for weight loss?

Do you have a specific date by which you would like to reach your long-term goal? *If not, I highly recommend you link your goal to an event such as a holiday, a birthday or a class reunion.*

EATING HABITS

Do you believe you mostly eat healthy foods?

What is the most vulnerable time of day for you when it comes to snacking or overeating?

How much fruit do you eat each day? When? What varieties? And is it dried, fresh, canned, frozen or a combination?

How many vegetable servings do you eat each day, and what types do you typically consume?

What is your biggest vice?
(dessert, French fries, chocolate, alcohol, soda, chips, etc.)

EXERCISE HABITS

Do you feel your cardiovascular endurance is good, or do you get out of breath easily?

How many days a week do you exercise for at least 30 minutes?

Does your body feel toned? Where? What areas do you want to improve?

OVERALL ENERGY & HEALTH

How much plain water do you drink daily?

Do you normally feel energized throughout the day? Do you get hungry or tired in the afternoon after lunch?

How many days of the week do you drink alcohol, and how many drinks do you consume at once?

What are you most proud of about your body? *Any feature counts, including luscious lips!*

How many hours of sleep do you get each night, on average?

MEASUREMENTS

Pants size:

Dress size:

Shirt size:

Measure the smallest part of your waist:

Measure around the largest part of your butt:

Measure the largest part around your thighs:

Measure across hip bones and around your tush:

GOALS

Now that you've answered some basic fitness and nutrition questions, let's identify your personal health goals.

Eating Habits: *(what specific changes do you want to make to improve your overall health?)*

Exercise frequency: *(how many days/week?)*

Long-term weight goal:

21-Day weight loss goal:

Week One Mini-Goal

Week Two Mini-Goal:

Week Three Mini-Goal:

Beyond 21 Days Goal: *(how do you want to feel and look?)*

Rules of Purposeful Engagement

The secret to leading a life of greater health and purpose lies in action—engaging in activities that strengthen your body, your spirit, your mental fitness and your desire to live the life God intended you to live.

Cultivate good habits so they become a part of who you are and how you live out your days. Parents enforce some of the habits we learn early in life, like brushing your teeth and washing your hands. Now that you are in charge, learn which habits will carry you towards the energy you want to exude and the happy life you want to foster.

As you begin this journey, please make a deal with yourself to commit to the following rules. They are the foundation to your being successful.

1. Weigh yourself as soon as you wake up, after you've gone to the bathroom and before eating or drinking anything. You can do this . . . weigh yourself naked. We need to know the point from which you are starting. As you work through the 21-Day Action Plan, strive to weigh yourself this way at least once a week. If you prefer to get on the scale more often, that's fine. I encourage you to keep track of your progress. After this challenge ends, get on the scale once a week to stay motivated and to avoid any surprise weight gain. After all, it's far easier to lose two pounds than 10.
2. Drink 90 or more ounces of water each day as recommended on page 19. Drink a glass of water right before each meal and, if you're still hungry after eating, drink 12 gulps of water and immediately brush your teeth. You *will* lose weight simply by doing this. Hydration is good for your heart and muscles. Go to www.mollyshattuck.com for all of your hydration necessities, including BPA-free filtered and unfiltered water bottles, filtered pitchers and more.
3. Eat a minimum of five servings of fresh vegetables and fruits each day. Limit your consumption of packaged, processed foods that are loaded with salt, sugar and chemicals. They provide few nutritional/health benefits and are linked to the obesity epidemic and illnesses such as cardiovascular disease, diabetes and certain kinds of cancer. Follow my recommendations on what to consume by carefully reading *Eat REAL* (page 26) and by using the *Grocery List* (page 82) and *Make REAL Meals* (page 148) I've provided.

   Make it more difficult to eat junk by simply not buying it—that means keeping it out of your home, office and car. You'll also be surprised how much money you'll save.

4. Limit alcohol, soda and sports drinks since they tend to provide an initial *rush* followed by a crash and reduction in energy. These drinks are likely to cause you to eat more and gain weight. And furthermore, these drinks can also increase your risk of cancer. Moderation is key.
5. Pack nutritious, portable snacks such as a serving (12–15) of unsalted almonds or walnuts. When that unexpected moment of hunger strikes, you will be armed with a healthy option.
6. Update the Daily Log by recording your intake of water, consumption of vegetables and fruit, amount of exercise and hours of sleep each night.
7. Write down *everything* you consume, if one of your main goals is to lose weight. Logging your food and drink forces you to stop and think about what you are putting into your mouth. This intentional action could decrease your caloric intake.
8. Follow the exercise schedules on pages 93, 109 and 125. With the purchase of this book, you have *free* access to my DVD located at www.mollyshattuck.com. It offers the **Full Body Strengthening** piece (21 minutes), **Full Body Stretch** (15 minutes) as well as the **Cardio Dance Ensemble** (45 minutes), which includes squats, lunges and kicks. Get your kids moving, too, in the **Workout with Kids** in which I demonstrate exercise with my children!

   I designed the work-outs to be interval-training exercises. Your heart rate fluctuates throughout the routines, and nearly every aerobic move focuses on your core (if you maintain good posture and form). If these exercises are done consistently, you will feel sexier and improve the shape of your legs, arms, butt and core as your muscles become more defined. Keep in mind that the exercises become easier over time.
9. Always warm up for five minutes before exercising begins (jumping jacks, jump rope, dance, etc.) and be sure to cool down and stretch after a workout. Walking is an excellent way to cool down, but also be sure to stretch your muscles!
10. Choose to move each day, even if you don't have time to exercise the recommended minimum of 30 minutes all at once. Do 10 minutes in the morning and 20 minutes in the evening. You'll get the same benefit by doing the exercises in phases.
11. Concentrate on the muscles you are using during each move throughout the workout. By being mindful and focusing on what you are doing, you'll see better results in a shorter period of time.
12. Sleep. Strive for 7–8 hours each night. There is now scientific proof that we eat fewer calories if we are well rested. As an added bonus, eye puffiness can significantly decrease.
13. Share your success by partnering with our Vibrant Living Community. Activate your participation in the 21-Day Action Plan by sending me an email with your start date to vibrantliving@mollyshattuck.com. You will begin receiving additional daily tips and suggestions to help you reach your goals. Also, "like" me on Facebook at the Molly Vibrant Living page for daily information related to health, food, exercise, volunteer opportunities and more.

I encourage you to share your successes with friends and family, and of course, with the Vibrant Living Community at www.mollyshattuck.com. You can also email us at vibrantliving@mollyshattuck.com.

Grocery List

It's a blessing—this bounty of fresh vegetables, fruits and wholesome ingredients that's now available to us!

Commit to making great choices for three weeks and see what new habits you can forge. Once you incorporate healthy food into your diet, eating well becomes a delight rather than a task or struggle. Have you been a junk food "addict" for years? You might be surprised how quickly you stop craving packaged, processed foods once you make a determined effort to eliminate them from your diet. You can teach your body to crave, accept or reject any food, flavor or sensation. Items loaded with sodium and chemicals start to lose their appeal after you've spent a few weeks enjoying a diet consisting primarily of whole foods and fresh ingredients.

Spice things up! Experiment with spices and unusual food combinations, discover the simple joys of local farmers' markets and try new varieties of vegetables and fruit. Let healthy living become your new lifestyle.

Food is the best source for obtaining vitamins and minerals. Some people may need vitamin supplements to meet their daily requirements, so be sure to consult a nutritionist or physician with specific questions about your individual nutrition needs.

The first step to healthy eating is making wholesome food readily available. Purge your kitchen of junk food, stock the fridge with fresh, in-season produce and have access to pantry staples you can easily retrieve for healthy recipes.

Don't feel you have to buy everything on the grocery list I've provided. It is meant to offer guidance and to help ensure you always have a wide range of healthy items at your disposal.

A FEW WORDS ABOUT LABELS

Remember to always read food labels. The U.S. Centers for Disease Control and Prevention found in a 2012 study that people who read food labels weigh almost nine pounds less than those who do not.[42]

Judge the quality of the food you are purchasing based on the ingredients, not the name on the package. Fewer ingredients tend to yield a better product if the main ingredient is listed first. If a product has ingredients you're not familiar with or can't even pronounce, don't buy it. It is probably loaded with chemicals that can *harm* rather than help your body.

Avoid packaged or prepared food with high amounts of salt, sugar and fat—calorie intake will vary by individual but, generally speaking, 10 percent or more of any of these items of daily value (%DV) is considered high, while 5 percent or less is considered low. Be careful to take the serving size into account when assessing the %DV of packaged food. For example, based on the %DV, one serving of a can of low-sodium tomato soup might provide an acceptable amount of salt. But, if you consume the entire can, you'll likely reach or exceed your daily allowance of sodium.

Be cautious of nutrition claims on labels. Many of these claims are *purely for marketing purposes* and are not indicative of a nutritionally sound product. "Reduced" and "low" have different meanings. "Reduced" means the product has less sodium, sugar, etc. than the original version, but that doesn't necessarily mean it is "low" in these substances according to the %DV established by the U.S. Food and Drug Administration. The word "organic" is also used on many packaged foods, but it does not imply the food has a high nutritional worth.

Remember to wash all produce thoroughly before eating and cooking to eliminate any residual pesticides or bacteria. All grains and beans should be rinsed well, removing any damaged items. A spray bottle is a great tool to have in the kitchen. Use it to hold salad dressings and oils for sensible control when flavoring foods.

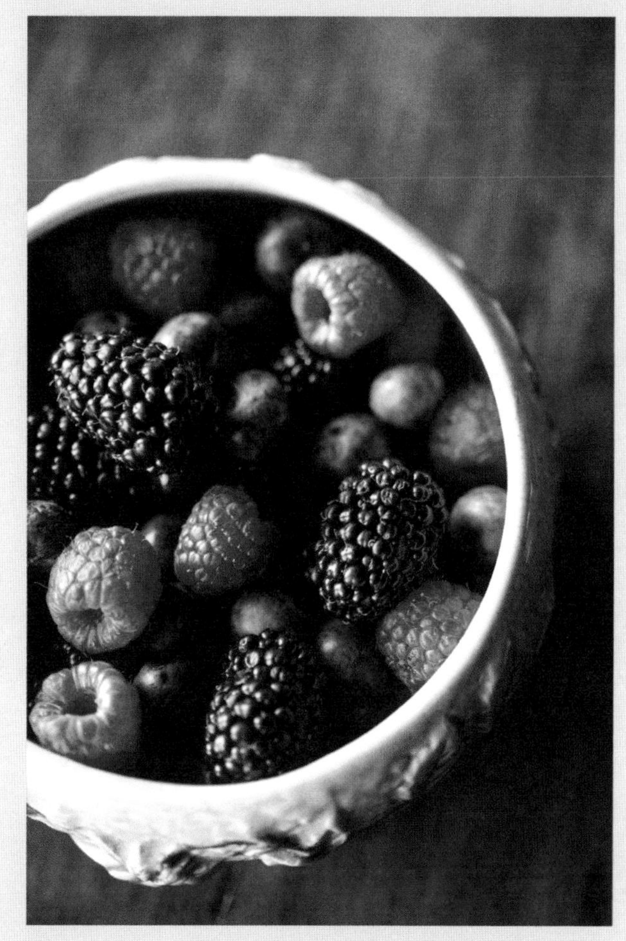

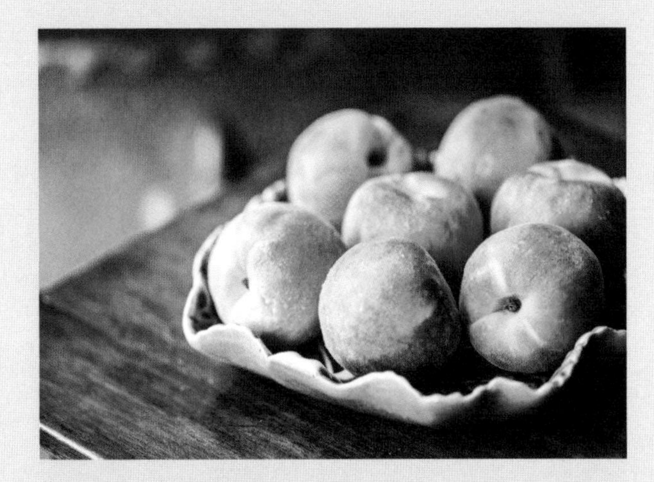

FRUIT

- ☐ Apple with skin
- ☐ Banana
- ☐ Berries: blackberries, blueberries, raspberries and strawberries
- ☐ Cantaloupe
- ☐ Pink and red grapefruit
- ☐ Red and purple grapes (remove stems, freeze and eat as a snack)
- ☐ Kiwi
- ☐ Oranges
- ☐ Papaya
- ☐ Watermelon
- ☐ Other seasonal fruit, such as fresh apricots, peaches and plums

VEGETABLES
(buy at farmers' market if possible)

- ☐ Asparagus
- ☐ Arugula
- ☐ Avocado (technically a fruit)
- ☐ Beets
- ☐ Bell peppers: red, yellow, green and orange
- ☐ Broccoli/broccolini
- ☐ Brussels sprouts
- ☐ Cabbage
- ☐ Cauliflower
- ☐ Carrots
- ☐ Celery
- ☐ Corn on the cob (limit serving size to one ear)
- ☐ Cucumbers
- ☐ Garlic
- ☐ Kale
- ☐ Peas (limit to one serving per day)
- ☐ Potatoes (limit to one serving per day)
- ☐ Spinach
- ☐ Squash
- ☐ Sweet potatoes
- ☐ Swiss chard
- ☐ Tomatoes (technically a fruit)
- ☐ Zucchini

PROTEIN

Non-Animal Sources

- [ ] Quinoa
- [ ] Hempseed (see **NUTS AND SEEDS**)

Animal Sources

- [ ] Eggs high in omega-3s (no difference between brown or white; organic and cage-free have nothing to do with nutrition)
- [ ] Organic turkey breast or whole turkey (for one main meal with leftovers for salad the next day and/or freezing)
- [ ] Fish/Shellfish (halibut, wild salmon, shrimp, etc.)
- [ ] Albacore white tuna fish in water
- [ ] Organic ground turkey breast
- [ ] Turkey bacon (1 slice per serving)
- [ ] Organic lean ground beef (limit consumption to one serving per week)
- [ ] Organic whole chicken (remove skin after baking) or skinless breasts

BEANS AND LEGUMES

- [ ] Adzuki beans
- [ ] Anasazi beans
- [ ] Black beans
- [ ] Black-eyed peas
- [ ] Chickpeas
- [ ] Edamame
- [ ] Fava beans
- [ ] Lentils
- [ ] Lima beans
- [ ] Red Kidney beans

WHOLE GRAINS

- [ ] Whole grain, high fiber cereal with no artificial sweeteners and fewer than 6 grams of sugar; fewer than 3 grams of fat; and less than 10% (DV) of sodium per serving: All Bran®, Special K®, Cheerios®, Total®, Kashi®
- [ ] Oatmeal: Old-Fashioned Quaker® Oats or steel cut oats
- [ ] Brown rice
- [ ] 100% whole wheat/grain bread or English muffins

DAIRY

- [ ] 1% organic milk
- [ ] Low-fat cottage cheese
- [ ] Plain Greek yogurt (add berries for more flavor)
- [ ] Cheese: part-skim mozzarella, feta, goat, Parmesan and Swiss (others should be reduced or low fat when possible or simply eat less of full fat)

NUTS AND SEEDS

- [ ] Unsalted almonds, cashews, walnuts: 12–15 per serving
- [ ] Pumpkin, flax and chia seeds: one Tbsp. per serving
- [ ] Simply Jif, Skippy Natural Creamy or nut butters such almond butter: one Tbsp. per serving

HEALTHY FATS

- [ ] Extra virgin olive oil: buy smaller size in a dark bottle and use within three months to maintain maximum nutritional value.
- [ ] 100% Avocado Oil

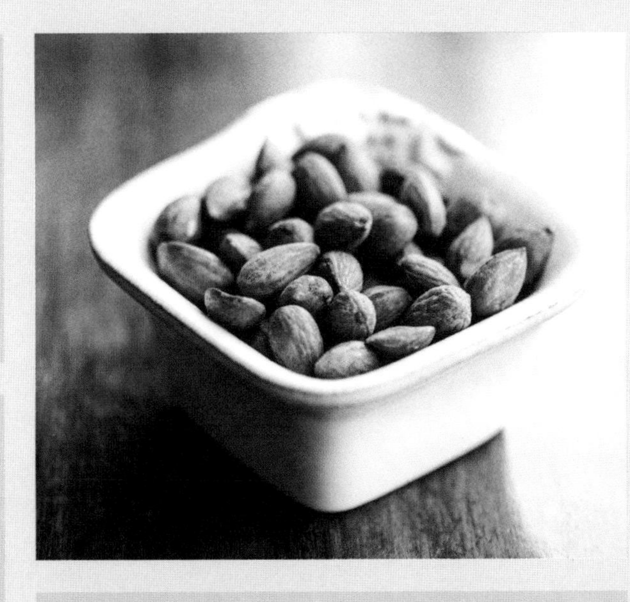

CONDIMENTS

- [ ] Dijon mustard
- [ ] Simply Heinz Ketchup
- [ ] Light mayonnaise (Hellmann's Light Mayonnaise is my favorite)
- [ ] Spray bottle for olive oil (use this to control the amount of oil added to your food when using to flavor)

SNACKS AND SWEETS

(limit to one serving per day)

- ☐ Skinny Pop® popcorn or plain kernels to pop on stovetop
- ☐ Fiber One® 90-calorie, Luna® and Special K® bars are my favorite (limit 1 per day)
- ☐ Kashi TLC Stoneground 7 Grain Crackers®
- ☐ Weight Watchers Giant Chocolate Fudge Ice Cream Bar®
- ☐ Skinny Cow Low Fat Ice Cream Sandwich®
- ☐ Strawberry Sorbet
- ☐ Dark chocolate: 70% cacao or higher (1–2 oz. per serving)
- ☐ York Miniatures® peppermint patties (1–2 per serving)
- ☐ Unsweetened applesauce (no artificial sweeteners)
- ☐ Roasted and unsalted soy nuts
- ☐ See *Make REAL Meals* (page 148) for more snack ideas.

TO BUY OR NOT BUY ORGANIC PRODUCE?

The Environmental Working Group states "The health benefits of a diet rich in fruits and vegetables outweigh the risks of pesticide exposure." We should, however, be aware of the foods that have the most pesticide residue (known as the Dirty Dozen Plus™) and when possible, buy the organic version. If you cannot afford the more expensive option (organic) of these fruits and vegetables, take extra care when rinsing the foods prior to eating, as you would even if it's labeled "organic." Below is the "dirty dozen."

15 FOODS MOST CONTAMINATED WITH PESTICIDES*

- Apples
- Celery
- Cherry tomatoes
- Cucumbers
- Grapes
- Hot peppers
- Nectarines—imported
- Peaches
- Potatoes
- Spinach
- Strawberries
- Sweet bell peppers
- Kale
- Collard greens
- Summer squash

*According to the Environmental Working Group, August, 2013

Dining Out Guide

Small changes can make a huge difference in creating healthier restaurant meals. Portion control is key, particularly when you are dining out, since serving sizes in U.S. restaurants are typically double the sizes of those in other countries. This phenomenon contributes to the high obesity rate in America, which currently hovers at 68% of people either obese or overweight.[43] These epidemic levels have caused a significant increase in heart disease, high blood pressure and diabetes.

Ultimately, *you* are the one who decides what goes into your mouth. And *you* can control what you eat, while marching towards your goals, without giving up the pleasure of dining out with friends and family.

MODERATION & KEEPING TAKE-OUT TO A MINIMUM

Dining out can be a relaxing and pleasurable break from the stress and routine of work, school or household chores. But *do it in moderation* and keep take-out meals to a minimum. Consider dining out a special treat and focus on the experience as a whole. Don't gobble your food. Eat slowly, being mindful of every bite, while you fully engage in your company and conversation. Choose an interesting restaurant—perhaps one with special cultural or historic significance—and take pleasure in your surroundings.

Keep in mind that eating out is not an invitation to pig out. Avoid the temptation to overindulge in super-sized meals by asking for a doggy bag when you place your order. When the food arrives, immediately put half away for lunch or dinner the next day. Alternatively, consider sharing an entrée. You'll be proud of yourself as you push away from the table without being overly stuffed and feeling lethargic or regretful.

GETTING REAL ABOUT EATING OUT

Here are a few other suggestions that can help cut a surprising number of calories and still help you feel satisfied:

- To help control your appetite, drink 12-16 ounces of water before you walk into the restaurant.
- Ask for dressing and condiments on the side. *You* should be the one adding the high-calorie, fat or sugary items such as mayonnaise and ketchup to your meal.
- Dress salad with olive oil vinaigrette ordered on the side. Dip your fork in the dressing before each bite instead of pouring it over your greens.
- Always request *no salt* on your food, opting instead to add it at your discretion if you think it's absolutely necessary.
- Choose tomato/marinara instead of meat or cream sauce if you're ordering pasta and add vegetables to it, naturally downsizing the amount of pasta in the dish. Remove the temptation to eat that huge portion by packaging half of it as soon as it is placed in front of you—don't tempt yourself to keep eating.
- When eating a sandwich trade out a slice of bread for a bed of lettuce or thick slice of tomato. One slice of homemade bread is delicious on its own but you really don't taste it on a sandwich and can easily do without the extra calories. If you still want bread with your meal but there are no homemade or whole-grain options, a light multi-grain English muffin is a good substitute.
- If you want ice cream, order the smallest size offered. Skip the waffle cone and toppings.
- Exchange blue cheese for feta or Parmesan and ask for it on the side. Adding it in small amounts may help you consume less than you would if you allow the restaurant to dictate the portion. Do the same if you want bacon on a salad; ask for it on the side and add a small amount for flavor.
- Order green salads as your meal—with a lean protein such as grilled fish or chicken.
- If the restaurant offers bread, treat yourself to one piece with a teaspoon or pat of butter, then *stop*.
- Don't use food as a trophy. Instead, celebrate your milestones by saving up for a vacation, buying a new pair of jeans or scheduling a massage.
- Start your meal with a salad loaded with veggies if you're not having one as the main dish. It will help satisfy your hunger more quickly.
- Order an appetizer portion of a main dish instead of the full-size version.
- If you want dessert, order fruit or sorbet.

Prep List

Before you dedicate yourself to your 21-Day Action Plan, gear up for success by doing the following:

- [ ] Check with your doctor before beginning any new exercise program. If you have any medical-related or physical limitations, share them with your doctor prior to beginning the 21-Day Action Plan. If you feel pain during any physical activity, stop what you're doing and stretch. Only begin again if you feel strong enough to do so.
- [ ] Buy a 30- to 34-ounce reusable, BPA-free water bottle and use it throughout the day. This is an investment in your health. If your home drinking water is not safe, go to www.mollyshattuck.com for filtered bottles and pitchers.
- [ ] Schedule workouts (See pages 93, 109 and 125 for Exercise Schedules) and bedtime on your calendar.
- [ ] Toss out processed, fat- and sugar-laden foods and beverages. Restock your pantry and fridge with whole, unprocessed foods—namely fruits, vegeta-bles, lean protein, beans, nuts, seeds and spices. Shop for healthy food options using the *Grocery List* (page 82).
- [ ] Plan meals and snacks for the week. Purposefully, write down what you're going to make for breakfast, lunch and dinner, then grocery shop for what you need for the week.
- [ ] Review all four sections of The Vibrant Living Workout DVD (available for *free* on the website when you activate your participation) so you have a general sense of what to expect when you're using it, as I recommend in the *Exercise Schedule* for each day of the three weeks.
- [ ] Complete the *Personal Goals* and share what you want with the Vibrant Living Community at www.mollyshattuck.com for personal advice about your goals. All information you share directly with me is kept confidential.
- [ ] Activate participation in this 21-Day Action Plan by visiting www.mollyshattuck.com and click on *Activate 21-Day Action Plan now*.
- [ ] Prepare to weigh yourself as soon as you awaken in the morning, after going to the bathroom.

THE GOLDEN GIRLS

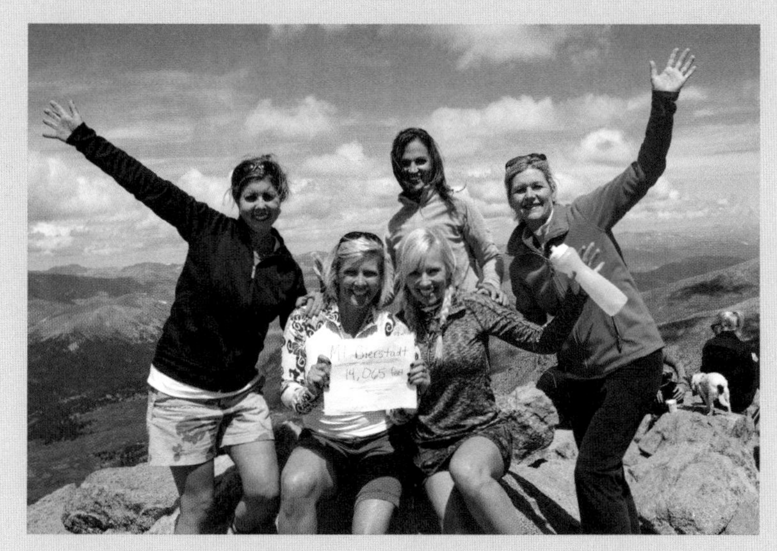

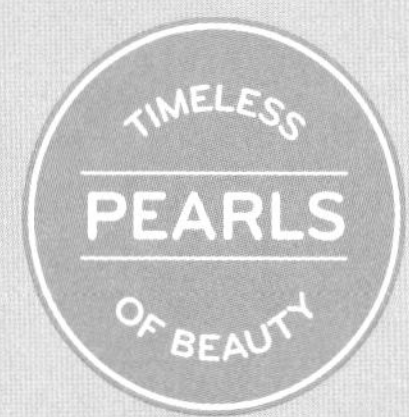

Look for this symbol throughout the Daily Log section!

I started an annual gathering many years ago with the Golden Girls, a close group of girlfriends. Yes, we watched "The Golden Girls" show when we were in college, laughing that we, too, would end up together as our time as wives and mothers wound down. Truly, we have been each other's virtuous circle, as loyal friends for nearly 30 years and some even longer. Through each joy in life and in its most challenging moments, we have provided an everlasting amount of support and comfort for one another. We all come together once a year for five days of camaraderie and endless life discussions. There are no boundaries or judgments, as we love each other for exactly who we are.

The Golden Girls' contribution to this book consists of 21 habits/tips for achieving and maintaining true beauty and wellness. We brainstormed the name and ideas during a recent hike to the summit of Mt. Bierdstadt, a 14,060 foot mountain in Colorado. That's when the Timeless Pearls of Beauty were born!

Daily Log

Here are recommendations for exercising during Week One of your 21-Day Action Plan. Weekly workouts include a combination of cardio, strength and interval training. In addition, I provide a bonus move (*Knock-Out Move of the Day*) each of the 21 days. Please do them in conjunction with this plan.

Since you are eligible for my free Vibrant Living Workout DVD by going to www.mollyshattuck.com and entering your book's SKU number, I have listed the option to use the DVD below. Be sure to schedule the exercise time on your calendar for each of the three weeks.

Always remember to warm up for five minutes before any workout and stretch while cooling down for a minimum of five minutes after every workout.

Before you begin, answer the following question:

What healthy lifestyle goal would you like to achieve over the next seven days?

FRONT PUSH-UP

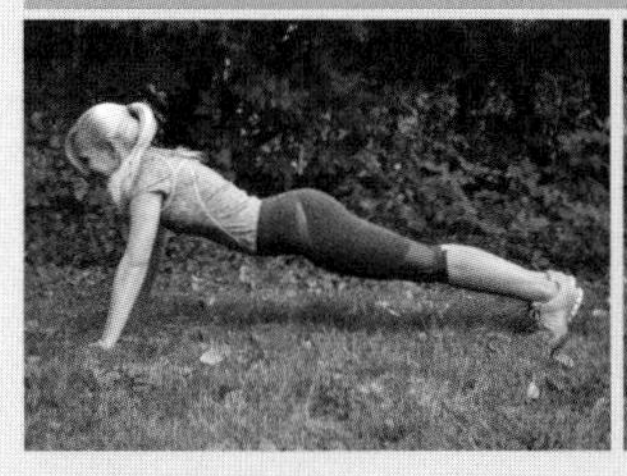

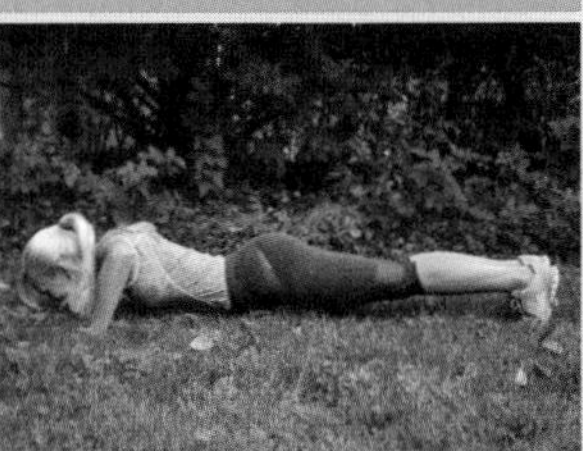

1. Get in position as shown above, balancing your weight on toes and hands while holding your tummy tight.
2. As you bend your arms to lower yourself to the floor, keep your neck straight and tummy in a firm position to prevent sagging towards the floor... then come up. Do not lift your tush in the air at any time.
3. Return to start position.

BACK PUSH-UP

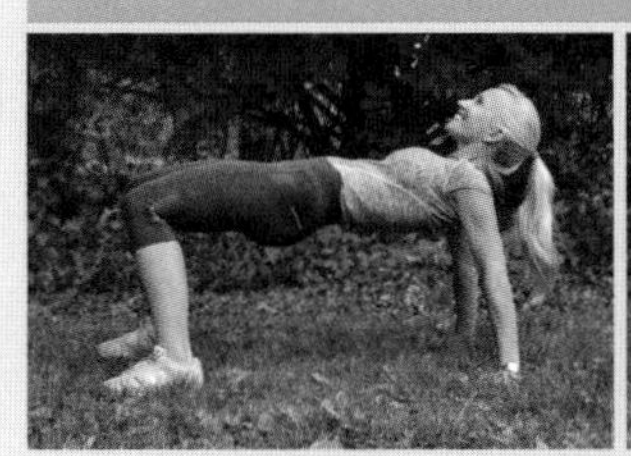

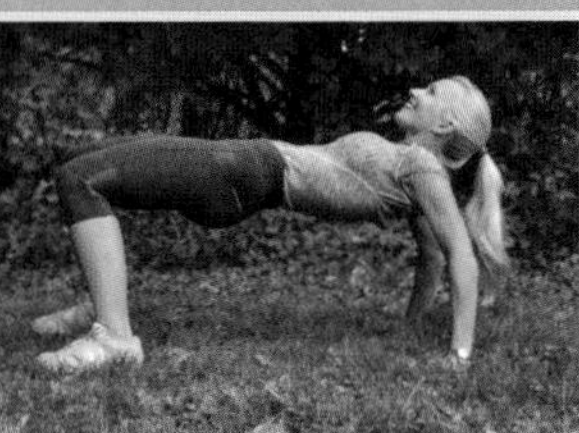

1. Get in position as shown above, balancing your weight on flat feet with straight arms, hands positioned toward lower body but slightly angled outward. Look out while keeping chin up and tush held high—do not let it sag.
2. Lower your arms by bending at elbows and keeping tush up... then return to straight arms. The move is ever so slight, but the muscles you use are significant.

EXERCISE SCHEDULE: Week One

DAY 1 Walk briskly for 5 minutes, stop and do 25 jumping jacks. Repeat combination for at least 30 minutes.
DVD OPTION: **Cardio Dance Ensemble** (45 minutes; includes warm-up, workout & stretching)

DAY 2 Jump rope for 3 minutes, do 25 front push-ups and 30 back push-ups (see image). Repeat combination three more times for a total of 100 front push-ups, 120 back push-ups and 12 minutes of jump rope.
DVD OPTION: **Full Body Strengthening** (21 minutes)

DAY 3 Cardio of your choice for at least 30 minutes (swim, bike, brisk walk, jog, rollerblade—do the moves at a pace that increases your heart rate).
DVD OPTION: **Cardio Dance Ensemble**

DAY 4 Hop kicks (hop with alternating leg kicks) for 3 minutes, 25 front push-ups and 30 back push-ups. Repeat combination three more times for a total of 100 front push-ups, 120 back-ups and 12 minutes of hop kicks.
DVD OPTION: **Full Body Strengthening**

DAY 5 Gentle walk for 20 minutes or longer.
No DVD option

DAY 6 Jog or dance in place to music for 3 minutes, 25 front push-ups and 30 back push-ups. Repeat combination three more times for a total of 100 front push-ups, 120 back-ups and 12 minutes of jogging or dancing.
DVD OPTION: **Full Body Strengthening**

DAY 7 Interval walk-run for 30 minutes. (Walk for 4 minutes, run for 2 minutes) Repeat combination for a minimum of 30 minutes.
DVD OPTION: **Cardio Dance Ensemble**

1

"Being in shape is not about being skinny; it's about being strong, feeling sexy and living out loud."

MOLLY SHATTUCK

The better our self-image, the more empowered we will be to achieve any goal. We are independent women and men who embrace work, family life and our communities, and we need physical strength to do it. Daily exercise and nutritious food charge our bodies with the fuel we need to get strong.

- Take a photo of yourself wearing a swimsuit or undergarments and tape it in the back of this book. Seeing what you look like on the day you begin the program can help motivate you to be more committed to it. Repeat this action after 21 days and compare photos. Progress motivates you to continue repeating healthy habits.
- If you haven't scheduled workouts and bedtime on your calendar, do it today!
- Try on a pair of jeans or dress in your closet you want to be able to wear, and keep them/it out as motivation. You'll be looking fabulous in this item very soon!
- Eat fresh fruit at breakfast and as an afternoon snack. Eat fresh vegetables at lunch, for a snack and at least two servings at dinner. Even try adding kale and spinach to a morning smoothie! The veggies and fruit help keep blood clean and inflammation down. Do this every day.

♥ Save trees by paying bills online. Go to PayItGreen.org to calculate how much water, oil and greenhouse gas you'll conserve annually by going digital. If 2 percent more U.S.households switched to electronic statements, we'd save nearly 200,000 trees each year.

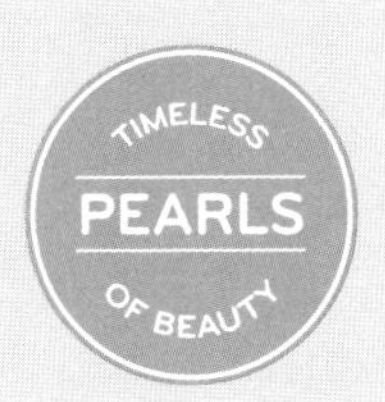

End your shower with a cold rinse. Instant tightened skin and shiny hair!

KNOCK-OUT MOVE OF THE DAY

TUSH LIFTER

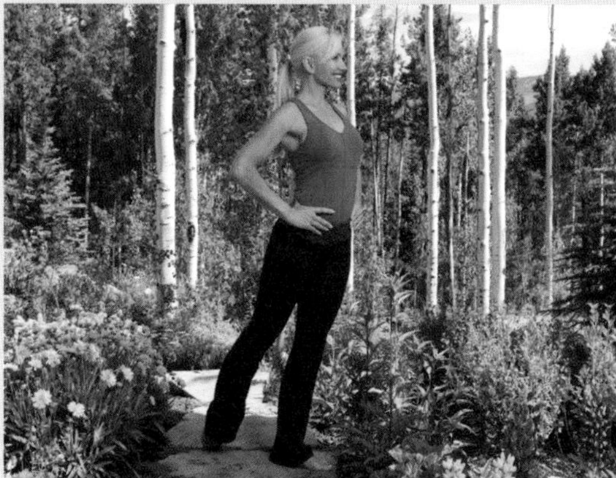

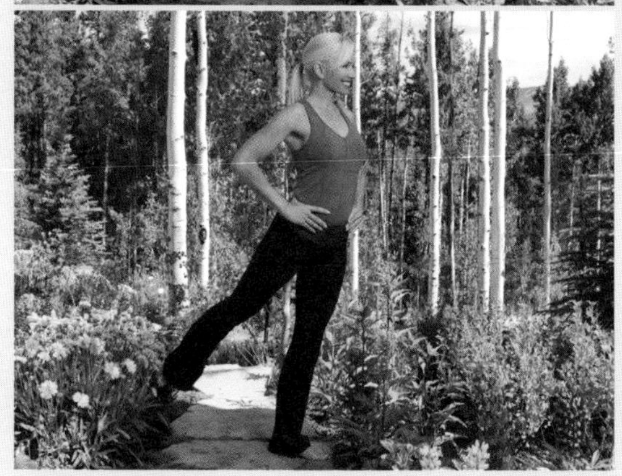

1. Stand straight on one leg with toe angled to corner. Keep your shoulders back, chin up and tush tucked under. Point your other leg back, toes pointed and knee angled to side.
2. Keeping your body straight, lift and lower the back leg.
3. Repeat 24 times and switch legs. Do four sets.

TODAY'S LOG

STARTING WEIGHT

EXERCISE

Description	Length of time

VEGETABLES AND FRUIT Strive for 5 servings.

1	4
2	5
3	

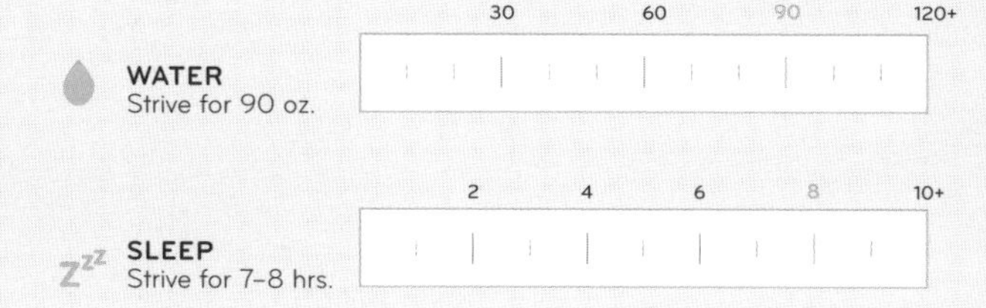

2

"Attitude is the paintbrush to life, as it can color any situation."

ANN TURNAGE

Focusing on what's good in any situation can completely change how you deal with a conflict.

- Visualize how you want to feel and what you want to look like at the end of 21 days . . . and beyond. Think energetic, lean and in control, starting today.
- Be selective about the clothes you keep in your closet. Remove items that support the "bulge" and are kind to weight gain. Never buy a size larger. Instead, drink more water, eat more REAL food, move your body every day and when you lose the weight, treat yourself to a new outfit!
- Commit to scheduled times to check technology throughout the day and otherwise turn your phone off. It will likely lessen stress in your life, and you will be more focused at the task at hand.
- Don't forget to complete your Daily Log. This task is designed to keep you on track and focused on what is good for your health.

♥ Hand-write notes to anyone who went out of their way to help or be nice to you this week.

Did you decide what you want your mini goal to be? If not, set it and write it on yesterday's page!

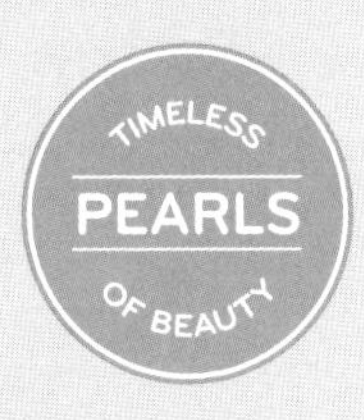

Rub a course loofah sponge for a minute or two in each spot of concern on your body (thighs, tush) during your shower.

KNOCK-OUT MOVE OF THE DAY

SCARECROW

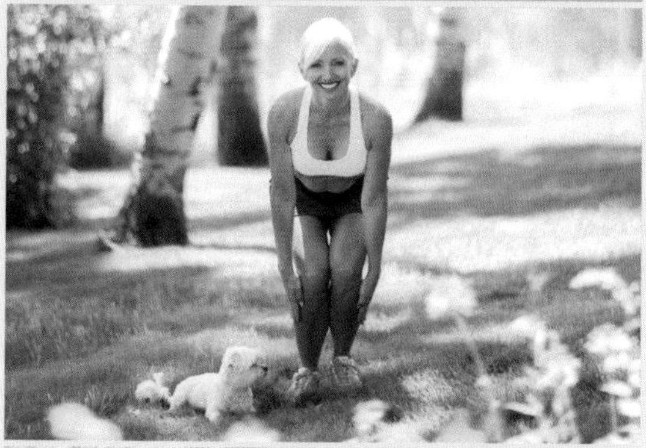

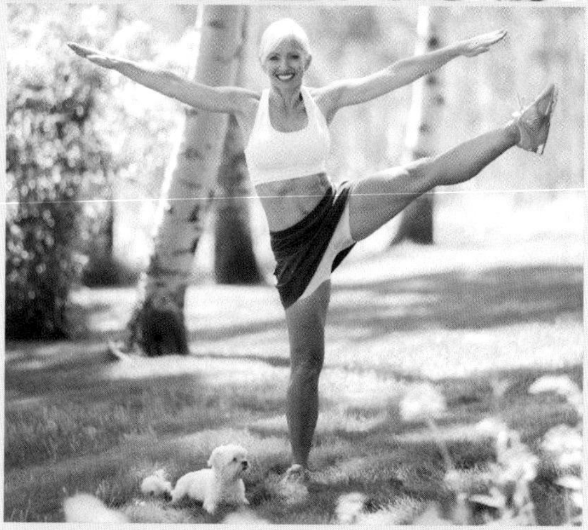

1. Stand with your legs together, arms by your side and knees bent.
2. Stand up while raising one leg—with toes pointed and both arms to the side. Return to starting position.
3. Repeat 12 times and switch legs. Do two sets for a total of 24 lifts on each leg.

TODAY'S LOG

EXERCISE

Description	Length of time

VEGETABLES AND FRUIT Strive for 5 servings.

1
2
3
4
5

WATER
Strive for 90 oz.

30 60 90 120+

SLEEP
Strive for 7–8 hrs.

2 4 6 8 10+

3

"Today is your day! Your mountain is waiting, so... get on your way!"

DR. SEUSS

This is an exciting time in your life. You are now taking charge of your health and body, and I'm thrilled for you. Stay positive! Making good decisions about water, eating and exercise creates daily successes. Everyone around you may start to notice your increased energy, so be open to the opportunities that come your way. You deserve them!

- Want to quickly diminish flab? The very best way is to do cardio intervals that alternate between bursts of heart-racing motions and periods of calmer movement. This kind of activity burns calories for hours after your workout.
- Never do the same exercise two days in row. Mix up your routine and be sure to follow the weekly exercise schedule I have provided.
- Prepare to cook for the week ahead. Plan what you will eat and when you will eat it using the *Make REAL Meals* (page 148) and the *Grocery List* (page 82) for inspiration and structure. Stock your fridge and freezer with healthy and delicious options.
- Don't forget to answer the questions I asked yesterday and share on the Vibrant Living Community. We want to help you and need your feedback to make recommendations.

♥ Participate in a military baby shower through Operation Shower http://operationshower.org. Learn how to make a "diaper cake" for the shower at mollyshattuck.com.

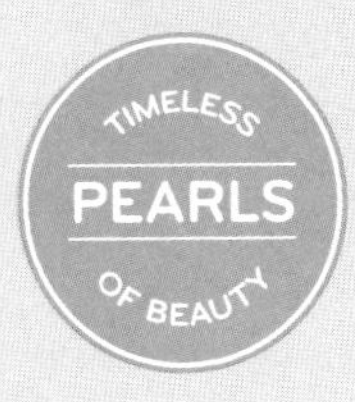

Wear a hat with a full brim to protect your entire face from damaging UVA rays whenever you're in the sun more than a half-hour.

KNOCK-OUT MOVE OF THE DAY

BLISS!

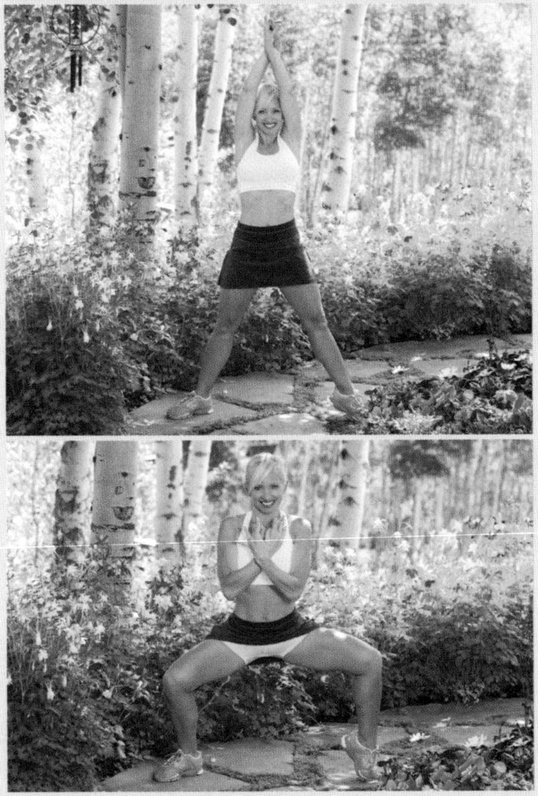

1. Stand with your legs in V-position, toes pointed to the corners and arms up and crossed over your head.
2. Lower your body to the squat position with your arms coming down and popping one toe with a heel lift. Return to start position, legs straight but keep your heel popped.
3. Repeat 12 times and switch legs. Do two sets for a total of 24 on each leg.

TODAY'S LOG

EXERCISE

Description	Length of time

VEGETABLES AND FRUIT Strive for 5 servings.

1
2
3
4
5

WATER
Strive for 90 oz.

30 60 90 120+

SLEEP
Strive for 7–8 hrs.

2 4 6 8 10+

4

"Throw away your excuses—for failing to exercise or make healthier food choices—and never look back. Live for today and the gift of tomorrow."

– MOLLY SHATTUCK

When history repeats itself in an unhealthy or negative way, be the one to break the pattern. Every positive decision you make is a success.

- Eliminate junk food from your diet and consume more fruit and vegetables. Doing this, together with drinking 90 ounces of water, can aid in immediate weight loss.
- Pause before you grab a handful of M&M's® or chips and drink 12 gulps of water. Walk away from the temptation and ask yourself if you really wanted the food or if it was more of a "ritual" that you now want to eliminate. Chances are you're thirsty, not hungry.
- Choose a mini dessert like a homemade chocolate chip cookie or peppermint patty if you really need something sweet after your meal. Desserts should be an occasional treat, not a daily one, and keep your portions small. Try fruit to satisfy your sweet tooth. Frozen grapes taste like candy and provide a shot of antioxidants.
- ♥ Advocate for animal welfare by volunteering your time, helping animals at the care centers, serving on rescue and response teams and organizing events to raise awareness and funds. Find a location near you by visiting: www.humanesociety.org/community/volunteers

Please answer the following questions and send your responses to the Vibrant Living Community at www.mollyshattuck.com.

1. Are you completing your Daily Log *every* day?
2. How much water did you drink on Days 1 to 3?
3. Have you noticed any changes in your energy level?
4. What is the biggest accomplishment you've had thus far in the 21-Day Action Plan?

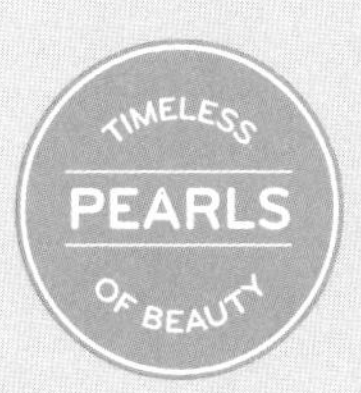

Apply coconut oil to dry hair, clip it up and let it sit for 30 minutes for silky hair. Shampoo as usual afterwards.

KNOCK-OUT MOVE OF THE DAY

LOWER LUNGE

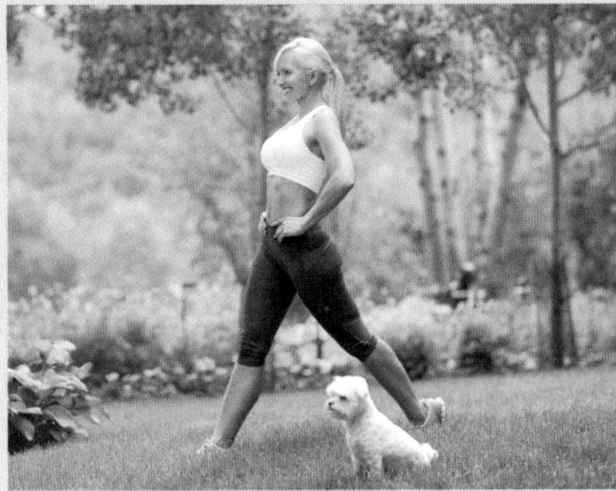

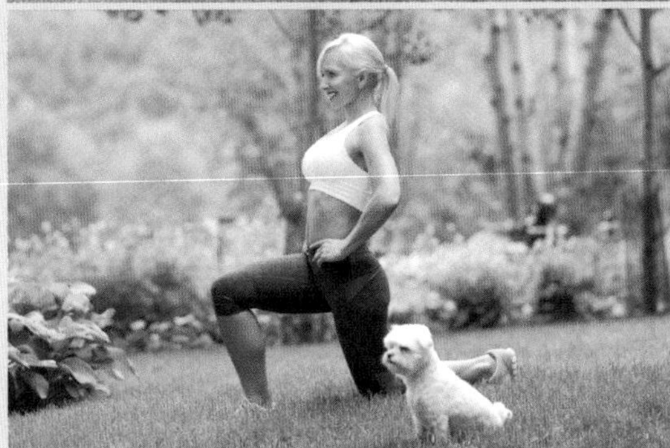

1. Stand with one leg straight in front, hands on hips, shoulders back and back leg straight, balancing on toe.
2. Lower your body by bending both legs then return to the original position. Be sure your front knee does not go over the ankle.
3. Repeat 12 times and switch legs. Do two sets for a total of 24 on each leg.

TODAY'S LOG

EXERCISE

Description	Length of time

VEGETABLES AND FRUIT Strive for 5 servings.

1	4
2	5
3	

WATER
Strive for 90 oz.

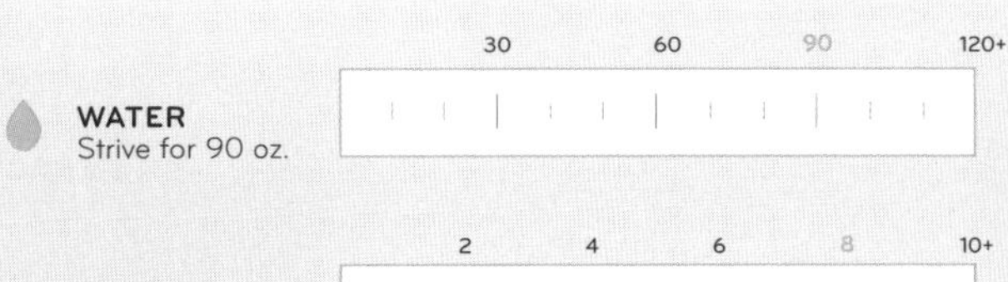

SLEEP
Strive for 7–8 hrs.

5

"The secret of change is to focus all of your energy, not on fighting the old, but on building the new."

SOCRATES

You are in total control of the individual choices you make for yourself each and every day. Fill your body with water and fresh produce. Take the time you used to spend picking up take-out to make your own at home. And choose to move throughout the day. No more procrastinating. Now is the time for *you*.

- Think "success." Visualize how you want to look and feel after losing weight and becoming healthier overall. Making changes is easier with clearly defined goals. It's now up to you to take action
- Start cooking your meals at home. Pack healthy snacks for when you know you're going to be on-the-go. Avoid the vending machines.
- If you're going to a party, you can enjoy yourself and still stick to your goals if you remain mindful of your choices. Make sure you aren't overly hungry when you arrive at the event and scope out the munchies for the healthiest options. Snack on vegetables rather than chips and use a small amount of dip. Have one cookie, not four, and then move away from the food. Make conversation, not eating, the focus of your evening.
- Drink 16 ounces of water before you arrive at any social event and at least a full glass for every hour you are there. These steps help you feel full so you don't overeat or consume too much alcohol.

♥ Shop at local farmers' markets to support local farms and merchants and fill your body with fresh produce.

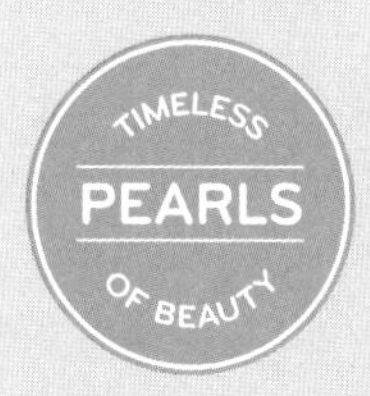

Dab pure vitamin E oil (capsule or liquid) around your eyes and lips every night to help reduce lines and other signs of aging.

KNOCK-OUT MOVE OF THE DAY

PUSH-OFF

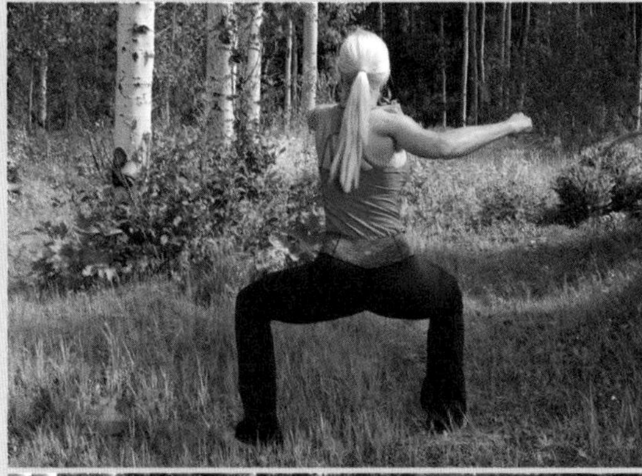

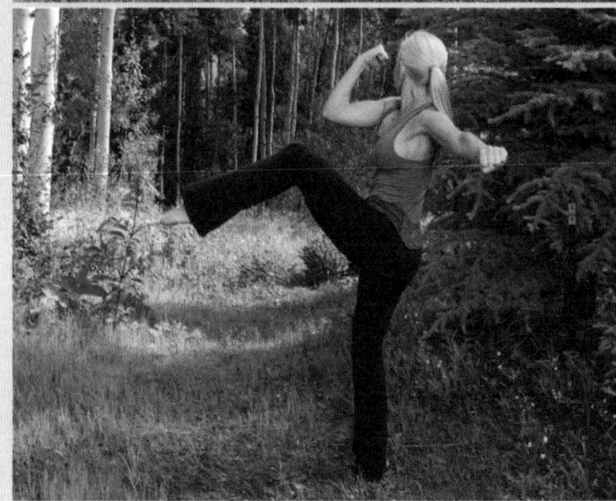

1. Stand in V position with your toes pointed to the corners and knees bent with arms held at shoulder level.
2. Twist your body coming up and touch the elbow to the knee of opposite leg, keeping toes pointed.
3. Repeat move 12 times and switch legs so that you twist in the opposite direction with other knee coming up. Do two sets for a total of 24 on each side.

TODAY'S LOG

EXERCISE

Description	Length of time

VEGETABLES AND FRUIT Strive for 5 servings.

1	4
2	5
3	

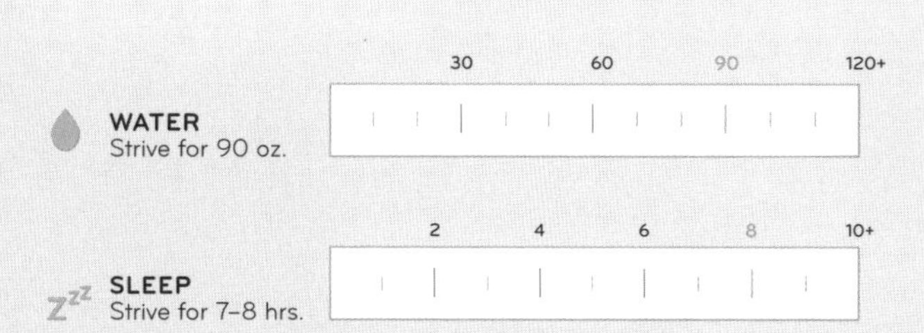

6

"The groundwork of all happiness is health."

LEIGH HUNT

When you are well rested, hydrated, eating healthy and exercising on a regular basis, you have a natural drive to improve every area of your life.

- Be sure to keep breathing during exercise if you find yourself yawning. Medically, it may not be proven but I have witnessed a strong correlation between the two.
- Stretch before you go to bed at night and you may sleep more soundly.
- Reward yourself for getting healthy by scheduling a massage. They are known to relieve muscle tension and pain, and even reduce stress. If you're like me and don't always have time for a full hour, consider taking advantage of a mall or airport kiosk for a 10-minute rubdown. On vacation, book 80 minutes!

Have you noticed any improvement in the appearance of your skin?

Have you made progress consuming more water?

Have you weighed yourself recently?

How many times have you exercised in the past seven days?

♥ Schedule a date to make and serve breakfast or lunch at your local Ronald McDonald House. These homes were created for families with loved ones who have a serious medical condition, requiring them to live outside their hometowns for an extended period of time. Find a Ronald McDonald House near you by visiting: www.rmhc.org/volunteer.

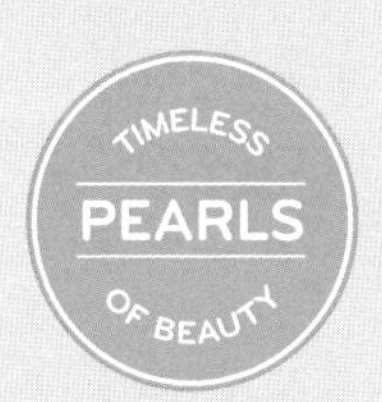

Smile and laugh every day. A steady dose of humor and laughter increases endorphins, dopamine and relaxation in your body.

KNOCK-OUT MOVE OF THE DAY

REVERSE HIKER

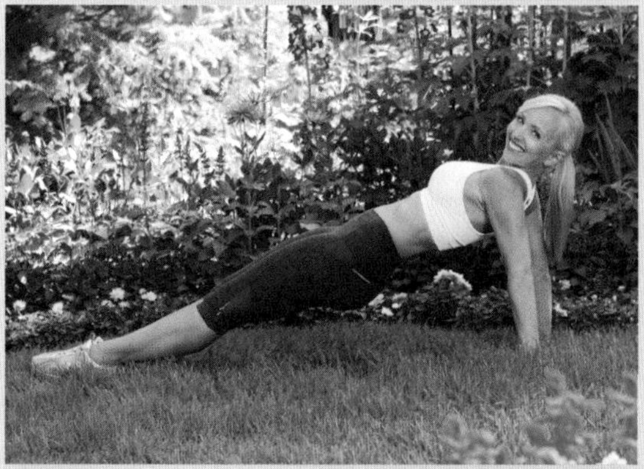

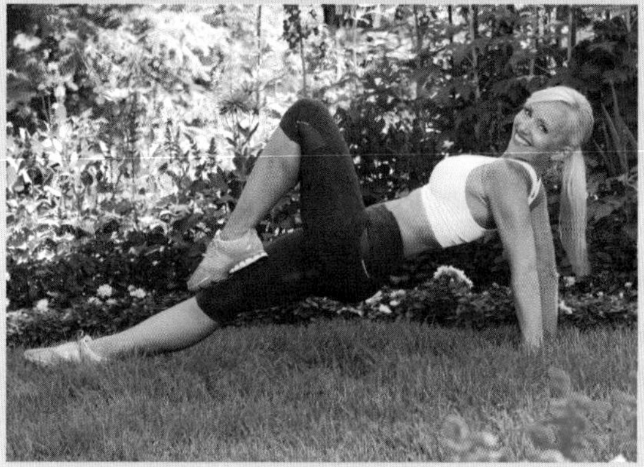

1. Position your body with straight arms and legs, your hands pointed toward feet and your butt held high.
2. Raise one leg with toes pointed to the knee of opposite leg while keeping your butt held high toward the sky.
3. Return to the start position and repeat 12 times then switch legs. Do two sets for a total of 24 on each side.

TODAY'S LOG

EXERCISE

Description	Length of time

VEGETABLES AND FRUIT Strive for 5 servings.

1	4
2	5
3	

WATER
Strive for 90 oz.

30 60 90 120+

SLEEP
Strive for 7–8 hrs.

2 4 6 8 10+

7

"Every goal begins with hope, and it's up to you to take action."

MOLLY SHATTUCK

Every day you have the choice to drink more water, eat better, exercise and help more people. Make the right decisions to yield positive results.

- If you haven't scheduled your bedtime each night, do it now and stick to it. It's proven that getting sufficient sleep reduces stress and promotes a positive attitude and more active mind. When we are sleep deprived, we tend to consume more calories because it fogs the mind and interferes with your ability to distinguish the difference between hunger, hydration and the need for sleep.
- On the seventh day, God said "Let there be chocolate." Indulge intelligently when you're rewarding yourself with a bite or two of deliciously dark chocolate.
- Stay away from artificial sweeteners as studies have shown they disrupt your body's natural way of counting calories and you may end up consuming more calories overall.[44] Furthermore, avoid fat-free products, as fat is likely being replaced with artificial additives, preservatives and other chemicals.
- ♥ Donate blood or volunteer with the American Red Cross. The Red Cross always needs volunteers with various backgrounds, talents and skill levels to help families affected by disaster; to provide care to those suffering from illness; or to assist military families and veterans. For more information, visit: www.redcross.org/support/volunteer/need-to-know.

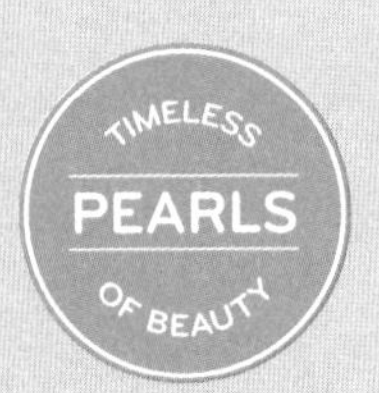

Don't clog your precious pores! Remove your makeup every night before bed.

KNOCK-OUT MOVE OF THE DAY

CROSS OVER

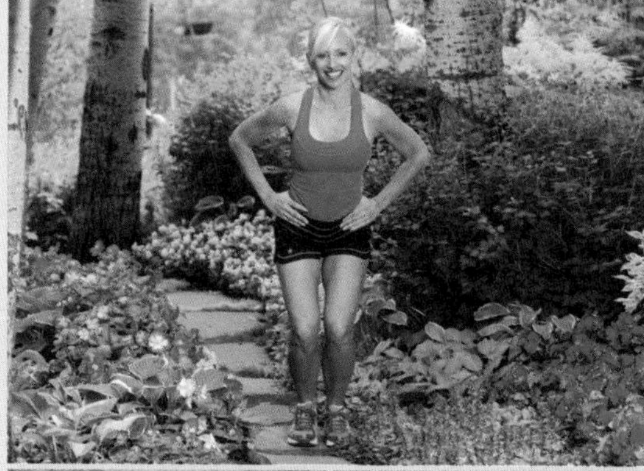

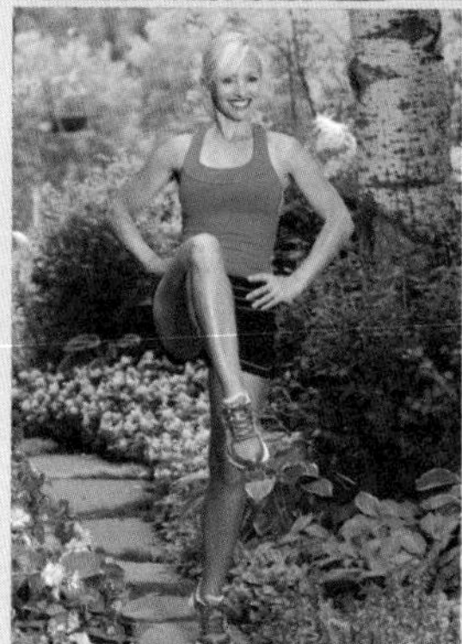

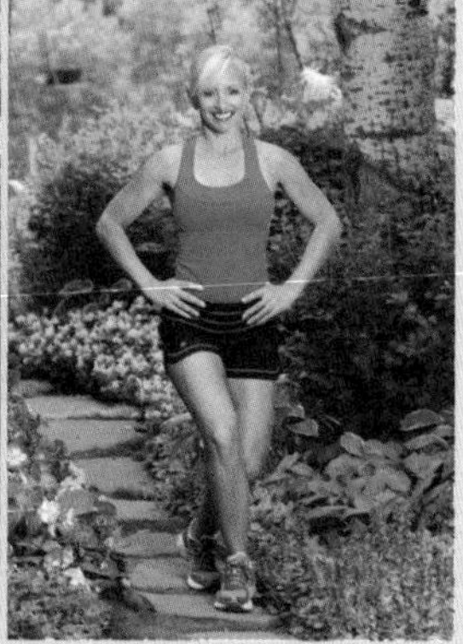

1. Starting with your legs together, hands on your hips, lower your body down.
2. Hop up with one leg raised and toes pointed (you will be on the ball of your foot doing the hop.)
3. Hop down, crossing the same leg over supporting leg.
4. Hop up, raising the same leg and return to starting position with legs together.
5. Repeat 24 times, then change legs.

TODAY'S LOG

EXERCISE

Description	Length of time

VEGETABLES AND FRUIT Strive for 5 servings.

1	4
2	5
3	

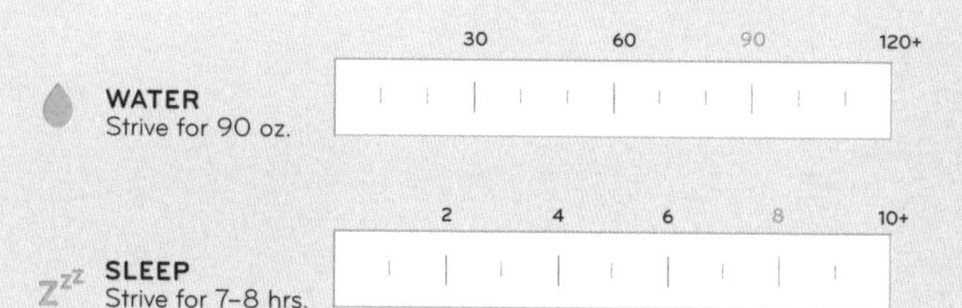

REFLECTIONS

Look back on your progress during Week One by recording your answers to these questions:

What healthy new habit is becoming easier each day?

In what way are you making better choices about food?

Are you more motivated to exercise each day and if so, why?

Are you getting 7–8 hours of sleep on average each night?

What action are you most proud of from the past week?

EXERCISE SCHEDULE: Week Two

DAY 8 Jump rope for 3 minutes, 25 front push-ups and 30 back push-ups. Repeat combination three more times for a total of 100 front push-ups, 120 back push-ups and 12 minutes of jumping rope.
DVD OPTION: **Full Body Strengthening**

DAY 9 Gentle walk, bike ride or swim for 20 minutes or longer.
No DVD option

DAY 10 15 squats (see image below), 25 jumping jacks and 25 jumping rope. Repeat combination three more times for a total of 60 squats, 100 jumping jacks, and 100 jumping rope.
DVD OPTION: **Cardio Dance Ensemble**

DAY 11 Jog in place with kicking your butt (bringing your heels to your seat) for 3 minutes, 25 front push-ups and 30 back push-ups. Repeat combination three more times for a total of 100 front push-ups, 120 back-ups and 12 minutes of jogging in place kicking your butt.
DVD OPTION: **Full Body Strengthening**

DAY 12 5 minute brisk walk, stop and do 25 jumping jacks, followed by 15 slow squats (1,000-1 going down; 1,000-2 coming up) and 15 fast squats. Repeat three more times for a total of 100 jumping jacks, 60 slow squats, 60 fast squats and 20 minutes of brisk walking.
DVD OPTION: **Cardio Dance Ensemble**

DAY 13 Gentle walk, hike or physical activity outdoors for 20 minutes or longer.
No DVD option

DAY 14 Hop kicks in place to music for 3 minutes, 25 front push-ups and 30 back push-ups. Repeat combination three more times for a total of 100 front push-ups, 120 back-ups and 12 minutes of hop kicks.
DVD OPTION: **Full Body Strengthening**

SQUAT

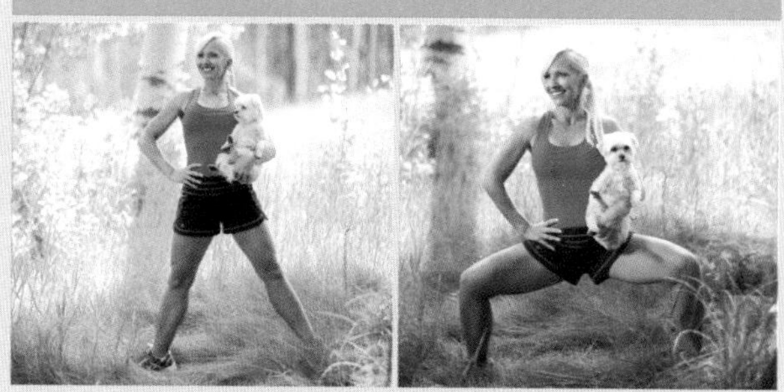

1. Stand in V position, your toes pointed to corner, hands on hips *or* holding your baby, dog or groceries.
2. Lower down to squat position and come back up.

8

"Take care of your body; it's the only place you have to live."

JIM ROHN

Good health is essential to each of us. It allows us to live the life we want for ourselves. Without it, we will have limits to what we can do.

- It's Week Two! Weigh yourself and record the weight in your Daily Log.
- Schedule your workouts on your calendar. Try to follow my recommended schedule but be realistic about your time. It's fine to divide a workout into smaller units to get it in: 15 minutes in the morning, 10 minutes at lunch and 15 minutes at night, for example.
- Plan your meals and snacks for this week, remembering that your body responds well to variety.
- Try on the jeans or dress you want to wear at the end of this 21-day period. Are you seeing a change? Applaud any progress and let it motivate you toward more success in the coming week.
- If you absolutely need dessert, the best option is a piece of fresh fruit or a home-baked goodie. Consider baking treats every other month and freezing them in single serving packages. It is tastier, healthier, less expensive and more convenient to grab a homemade chocolate chip cookie than to fill up on a store-bought version full of chemicals.

♥ Save the planet and money. If you don't have a bicycle, considering trying RentABikeNow.com, a network of more than 220 bikes across the country. And if you join Rails to Trails, you'll earn a coupon for your next rental.

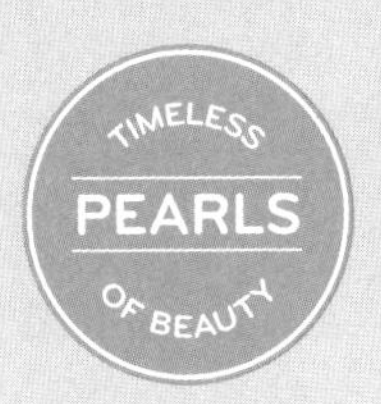

Moisturize daily (arms, tummy, legs) with body butter. Bath and Body Works' brand is the best!

KNOCK-OUT MOVE OF THE DAY

PULSE UP

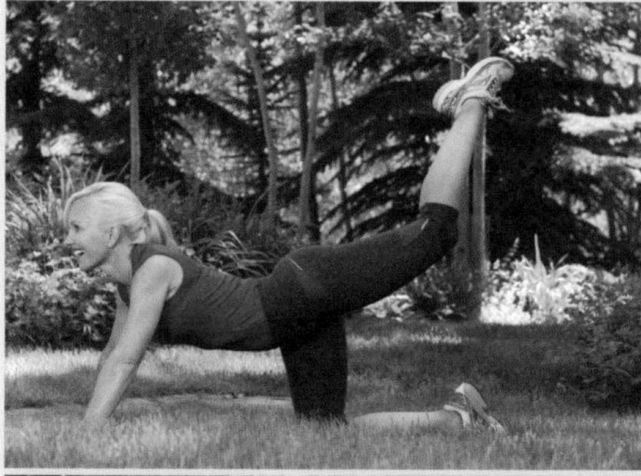

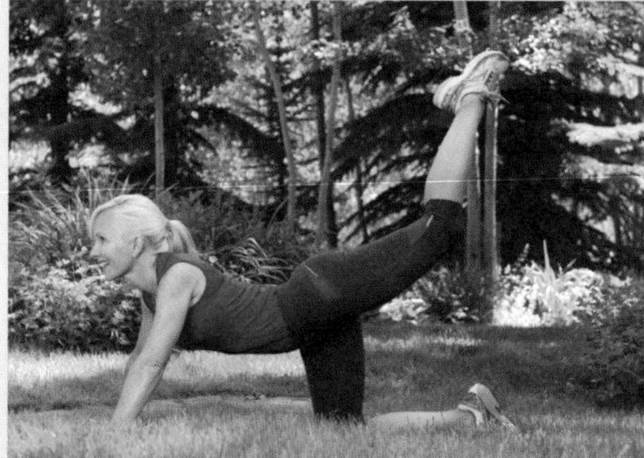

1. Get on both hands, one knee, and extend your other leg up with toes pointed.
2. Pulse the leg up and repeat 24 times.
3. Change sides and pulse your other leg 24 times.

TODAY'S LOG

CURRENT WEIGHT

EXERCISE

Description	Length of time

VEGETABLES AND FRUIT Strive for 5 servings.

1	4
2	5
3	

WATER
Strive for 90 oz.

30 60 90 120+

SLEEP
Strive for 7–8 hrs.

2 4 6 8 10+

9

"It's not selfish to love yourself, take care of yourself and to make your happiness a priority. It's necessary."

MANDY HALE

Ultimately, you are the only person responsible for your attitude and the way your clothes fit. Be accountable to yourself and welcome the opportunities that arise while you're making personal health a priority.

- Focus on what's good in your life. Embrace the people you love and reach out to those with whom you want to be in touch. Pick up the phone and call them or schedule a walk or lunch date. Make the time to contact the people who matter to you.
- Identify factors adding stress to your life and make an effort to negate them. Take time to breathe and think about out how to eliminate the stress that is having an unnecessary and negative impact on your life.
- No longer allow stress to drain your energy. Identify factors that add stress to your life and manage them by changing your response. For example, if you get stuck in traffic every morning, either leave earlier or, if you can't make that happen, stay calm by taking a deep breath and listening to music that makes you sing. If you're in a tense situation with another person, listen carefully and then share how you feel and make suggestions to help the situation.
- *Live intentionally!* You choose the life you want to have by setting goals and making plans to achieve them. *"Nobody gets to live life backwards. Look ahead . . . that is where your future lies."* — Ann Landers

♥ Help build a warm, safe and loving home through Habitat for Humanity. Bring a group to volunteer—of youth, women, veterans and more. To find out more, visit www.habitat.org/getinv/volunteer_programs.aspx.

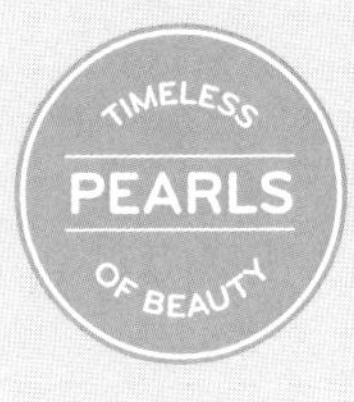

Use broad spectrum sunscreen—on every exposed inch of your body. Don't forget the tops of your toes, hands, ears, scalp and, of course, your face and nose. Reapply every hour in the sun.

KNOCK-OUT MOVE OF THE DAY

CROSS OVER LIFT

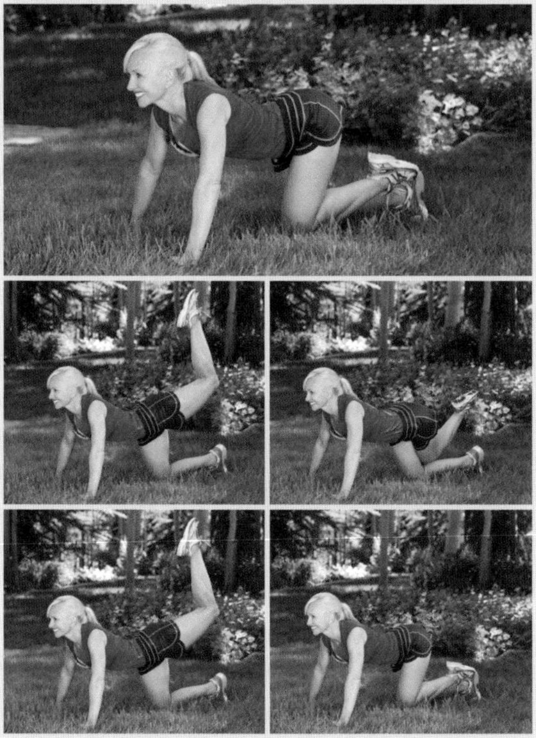

1. Get on your hands and one knee.
2. Lift one leg up with your toes pointed.
3. Lower your knee while crossing over your bottom leg.
4. Lift your leg with toes pointed.
5. Lower your leg back to start position. Repeat 12 times and switch legs.
6. Do two sets for a total of 24 on each leg.

TODAY'S LOG

EXERCISE

Description	Length of time

VEGETABLES AND FRUIT Strive for 5 servings.

1

2

3

4

5

WATER
Strive for 90 oz.

30 60 90 120+

SLEEP
Strive for 7–8 hrs.

2 4 6 8 10+

10

"Surround yourself with positive, supportive and encouraging people. Tell the world you're committed to getting healthy."

MOLLY SHATTUCK

When taking this action, you will discover many people want to get healthy and lose weight, too; you are motivating to others. Women, in particular, like being part of a tribe, as they gain strength and willpower from one another. But the same holds true for men. Be open to creating a tribe that suits your healthier lifestyle.

- Schedule your annual doctor/wellness appointments—with your general physician, gynecologist, dermatologist, dentist and eye doctor.
- Identify a positive habit you have formed this week, and share it with your friends and the Vibrant Living Community at www.mollyshattuck.com
- Schedule a walking date with a friend you haven't seen recently. You can have dinner, too, but only after you've enjoyed some exercise time together.
- If you have a television show you enjoy, watch it while doing some your *Knock-Out Move of the Day*, or a combination of them, then turn it off and pursue your other passions. In a recent study at University of Maryland, unhappy people were found to watch 20 percent more television that those who were content.

♥ Partner with the United Way to help mentor a child, teach someone to read, provide professional skills, or give healthy food to shelters and more. Find a United Way near you for a local project at apps.unitedway.org/myuw.

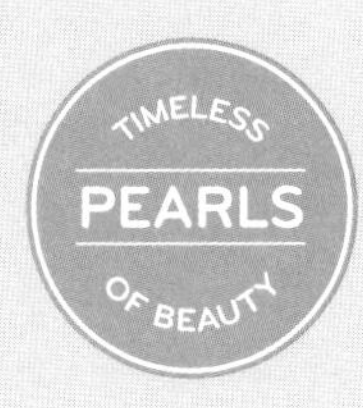

Be your own best cheerleader. Accentuate your positive qualities; wear clothes that fit and show off your curves! And don't bring attention to your flaws by mentioning them often to others.

KNOCK-OUT MOVE OF THE DAY

BLT

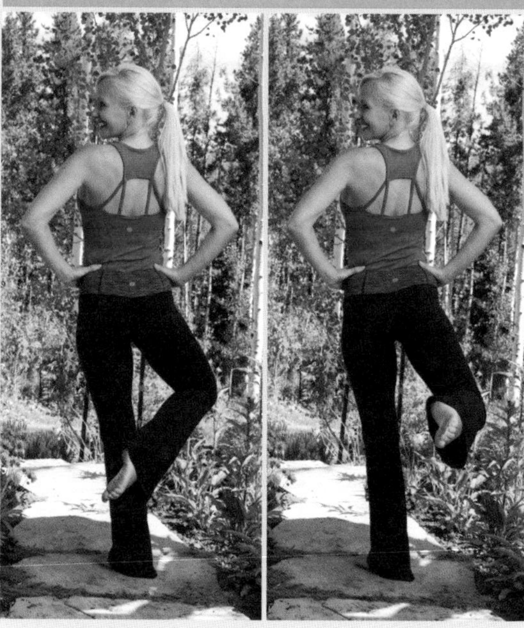

1. Stand straight on one leg, toes angled to corner. Keep your shoulders back, butt tucked under with your opposite leg pointed and crossed over the supporting leg.
2. Raise your back leg, while keeping your body still and shoulders back. Then lower it back to starting position.
3. Repeat 12 times then switch legs. Do two sets for a total of 24 on each leg. If needed, use a tree or chair for balance.

TODAY'S LOG

EXERCISE

Description	Length of time

VEGETABLES AND FRUIT Strive for 5 servings.

1
2
3
4
5

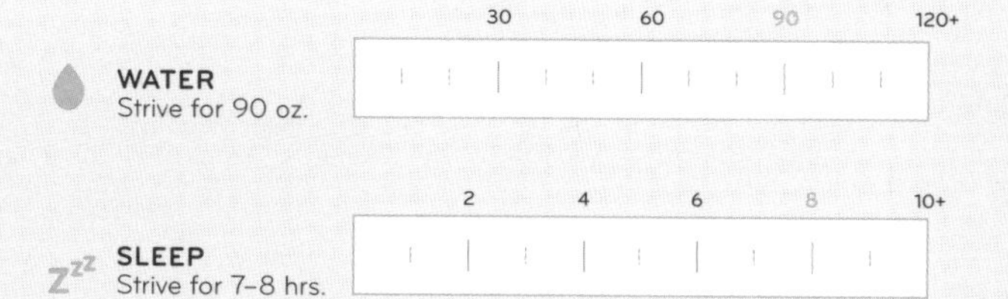

11

"The food you eat can be either the safest and most powerful form of medicine or the slowest form of poison."

ANN WIGMORE

Eating better foods, exercising, serving others and getting adequate hydration will have a profound impact on your life right now. And if you sustain this commitment to healthy living, you will be able to accomplish a number of great things you want for yourself.

- Minimize salt intake.
- Use herbs and spices to add more flavor to your food. Basil, black pepper, chili powder, cinnamon, cloves, cumin, garlic powder, ginger, oregano, red pepper, rosemary, sage, thyme and turmeric are rich in antioxidants and new evidence suggests they may boost your immune system and reduce inflammation, as well as help curb your hunger.[45] Check out the McCormick™ website for insightful information about spices: www.mccormick.com/SpicesForHealth.aspx.
- Add cinnamon to foods like oatmeal, whenever possible. It's a key antioxidant just like blueberries, and can help regulate blood sugar.
- Another reason to eat more fruit and vegetables: People who ate about five servings of produce daily scored better on memory tests than those who ate fewer, according to a study from Heinrich-Heine University in Dusseldof, Germany.

♥ Make a double batch of Vegetable Soup in *Making Simple REAL Meals* on page 163 and donate a batch to a homeless shelter or soup kitchen in your community.

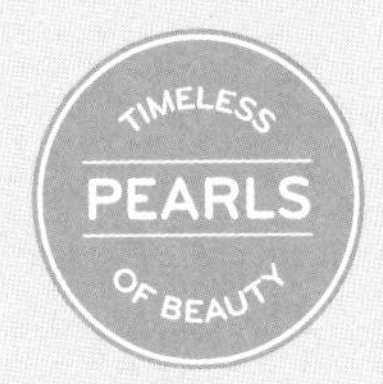

A recipe to exfoliate your body for radiant and ultra-smooth skin: Mix 1 cup dry oatmeal with ¼ cup honey and rub over dry skin. Rinse well and moisturize with body butter.

KNOCK-OUT MOVE OF THE DAY

SIDE HYDRANT

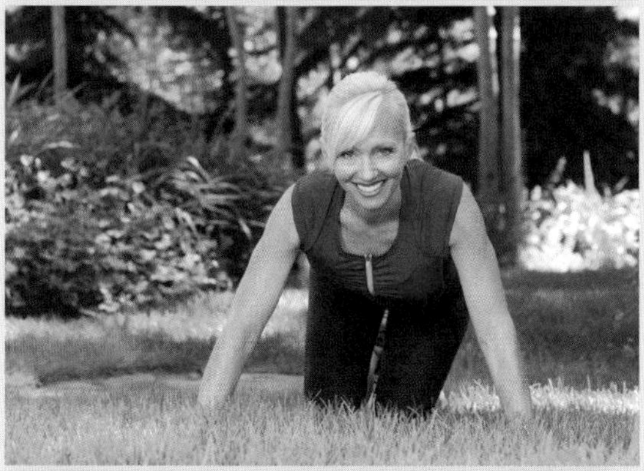

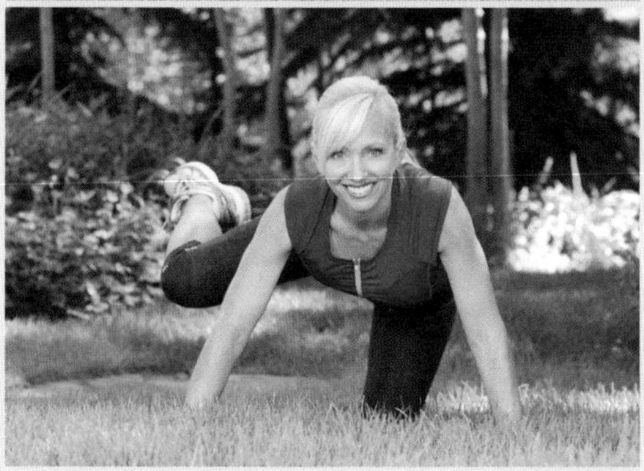

1. Get on your hands and one knee.
2. Lift one leg to the side, keeping your knee bent, toes pointed and lower it back to other leg.
3. Repeat 24 times and switch sides.

TODAY'S LOG

EXERCISE

Description	Length of time

VEGETABLES AND FRUIT Strive for 5 servings.

1	4
2	5
3	

WATER
Strive for 90 oz.

30 60 90 120+

SLEEP
Strive for 7–8 hrs.

2 4 6 8 10+

12

"Energy is the essence of life. Every day you decide how you're going to use it by knowing what you want and what it takes to reach that goal, and by maintaining focus."

OPRAH WINFREY

Turn your dreams into plans. As you become healthier and happier with your physical body, you will find a new zest for living and fulfilling your dreams.

- Pick up a hobby, like crocheting or bicycling, or learn how to do brain teaser puzzles like sudoku.
- Set four goals you want to accomplish this year. Write them down this weekend. Regardless of how big or small they are, you are more likely to reach them if you plan them out and commit to goals in writing. Many can be achieved with a little practice and training; others require ongoing dedication and focus. Create the life you want for yourself.
- Buy the ingredients for two or more of the dinner recipes in this book, beginning on page 160, and make them this weekend. Many of the suggested recipes freeze well so you can have healthy options available when you're short on time.

♥ Sponsor a care package for our dedicated military women and men through Operation USO Care Package. Visit here to learn how: www.uso.org/OUCP-donation-page-with-partner.aspx?LangType=1033.

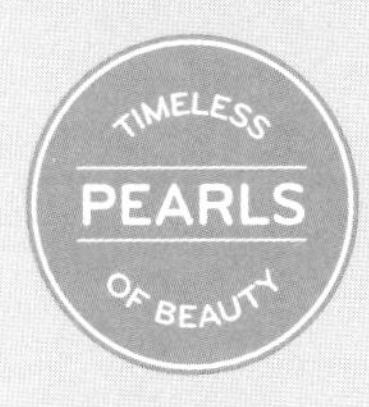

Reduce eye and leg puffiness *simultaneously*: Lie on your back with legs straight up against the wall, place ice cold cucumbers on your eyes and stay put for 15 minutes.

KNOCK-OUT MOVE OF THE DAY

STEP BACK LUNGE

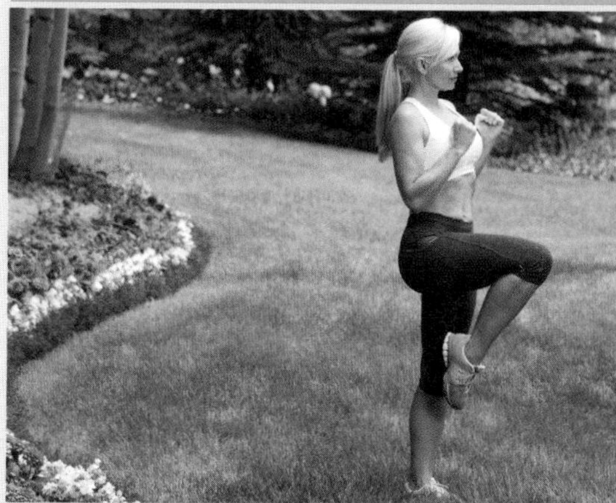

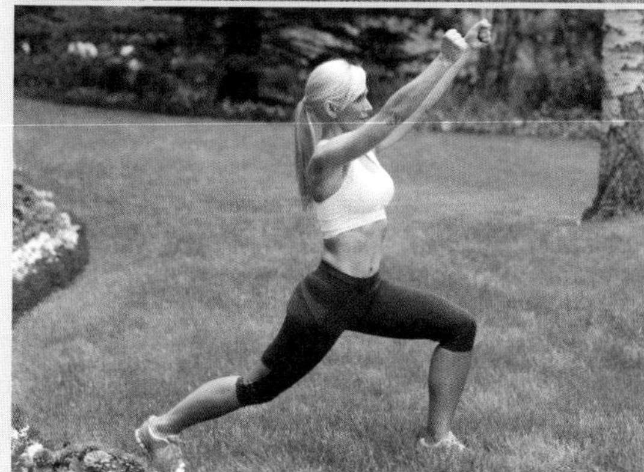

1. Stand on one leg with your shoulders back, arms bent, hands in fists and the other leg bent—with toes pointed—next to your supporting leg.
2. Lowering the supporting leg, step back. Put arms up and straight, at an angle. Return to start position and repeat 12 times, then switch legs. Work your way up to two sets for a total of 24 on each side.

TODAY'S LOG

EXERCISE

Description	Length of time

VEGETABLES AND FRUIT Strive for 5 servings.

1	4
2	5
3	

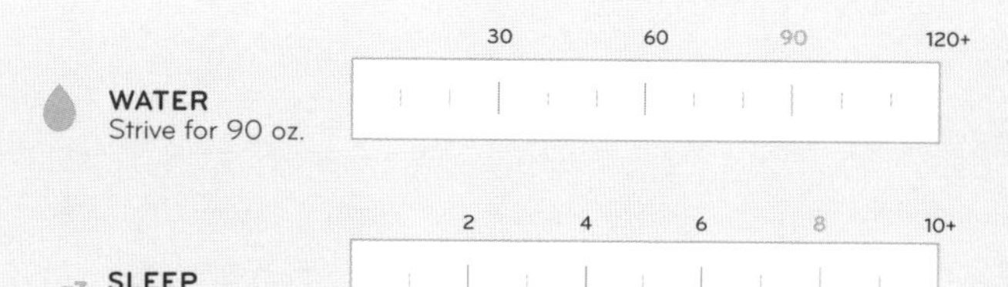

13 "Don't let others make decisions about what is best for you personally... you decide. It's *your* life."

MOLLY SHATTUCK

You are in control of your life, including what you eat and drink and whether you choose to exercise or not. Do your best to avoid being negatively influenced by others. They may love you dearly but fail to realize the **21-Day Action Plan** is your priority at this moment. Do this for *you*, and then let the perks of your higher energy and health spread to others.

- Work up a sweat when you exercise! When you're moving your body, get out of your comfort zone and push yourself to increase your heart rate. You should feel like you're working harder than you do when you're walking. It should be difficult to carry on a conversation. It's okay to be huffing and puffing on and off throughout your workout. Don't let a day go by without moving your body.
- To avoid osteoporosis, don't smoke, limit caffeine, and avoid excessive intake of alcohol, sugar and salt. Additionally, eat a diet rich in dark leafy greens, beans and legumes, and spend some unprotected time in the sun (no more than 30 minutes) before applying a broad spectrum sunscreen.
- Eat foods rich in antioxidants, like spinach, watermelon and tomatoes, to help repair cells damaged by the sun.

♥ "Create the Good" by working with your local AARP, which connects volunteers with service projects that best match your schedule and skills. To get involved, visit createthegood.org for more information.

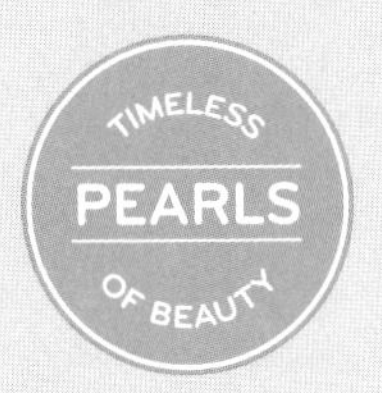

Calibrate your mind, body and spirit by taking pauses. Walk away from daily life for 15 minutes every day to do nothing.

KNOCK-OUT MOVE OF THE DAY

SIDE KICK

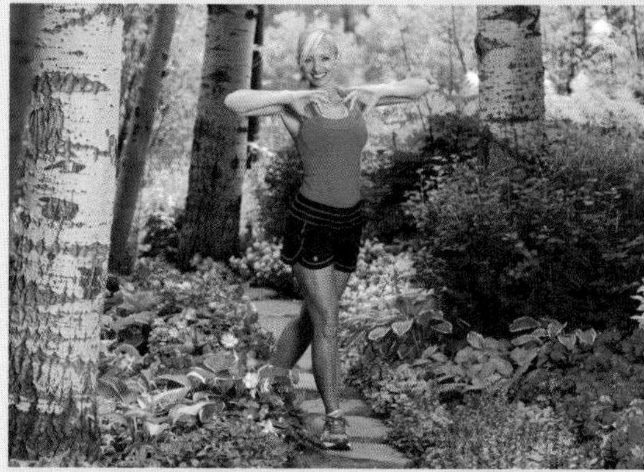

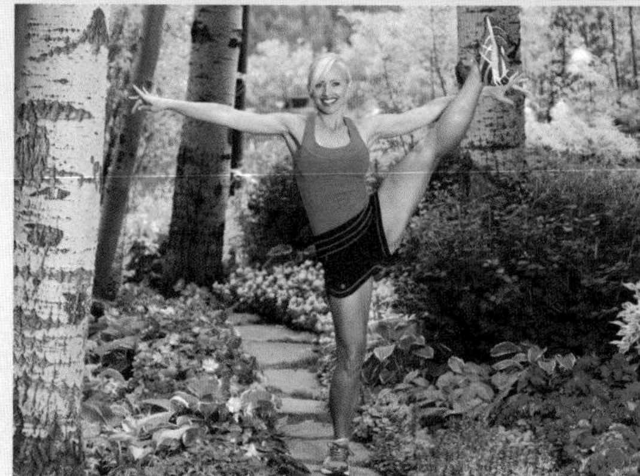

1. Cross one leg behind your supporting front leg with elbows pointed to sides.
2. Kick your back leg to the side with toes pointed. Return to starting position behind your front leg.
3. Repeat 12 times with that leg and switch sides to kick the other leg.

TODAY'S LOG

EXERCISE

Description	Length of time

VEGETABLES AND FRUIT Strive for 5 servings.

1	4
2	5
3	

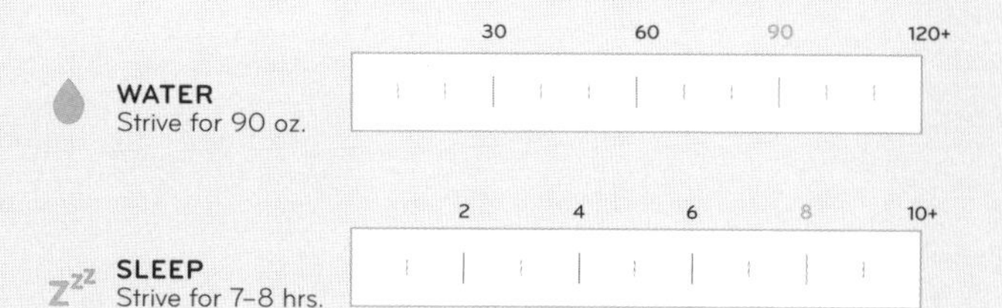

14 "Turn obstacles into opportunities for greatness."

MOLLY SHATTUCK

Unexpected situations and events happen in our lives. We have a choice about how to respond when something challenging occurs. We can surrender ourselves, become paralyzed by the event and let it define us, *or* we can focus on turning the unexpected into an opportunity. Move past mistakes and don't give up on your plan.

- Plan to take a one-hour brisk walk this week, in addition to your normally scheduled exercises. That single walk can extend your life by two hours![46]
- Fresh air is therapeutic, so be sure to get outside each and every day.
- Keep a pen and small notebook or pad of paper beside your bed. Before turning off the light, write down any "to do's" you have for the next day or ideas you would like to pursue. Writing a goal down on paper is the first step to making it happen. And this may be an excellent way to clear (and prepare) your mind for a more restful night of sleep. This has worked for me for years!
- Help unite the world by engaging with United Planet by visiting www.unitedplanet.org/take-action-more-united-planet.

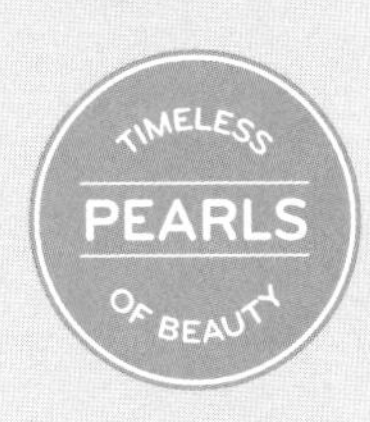

Pray every day for that which you are most grateful and for someone else who may need help.

KNOCK-OUT MOVE OF THE DAY

FROGGY

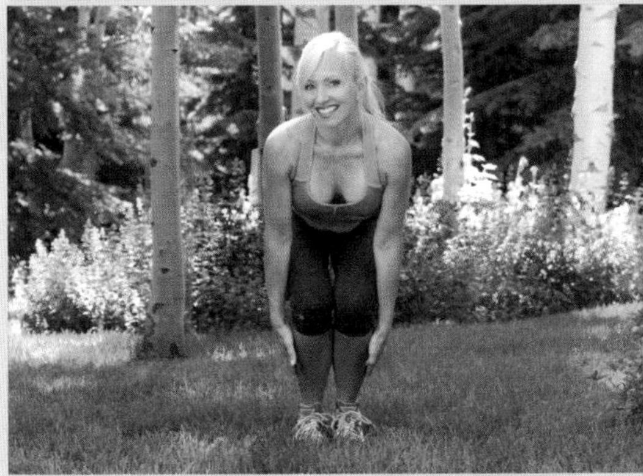

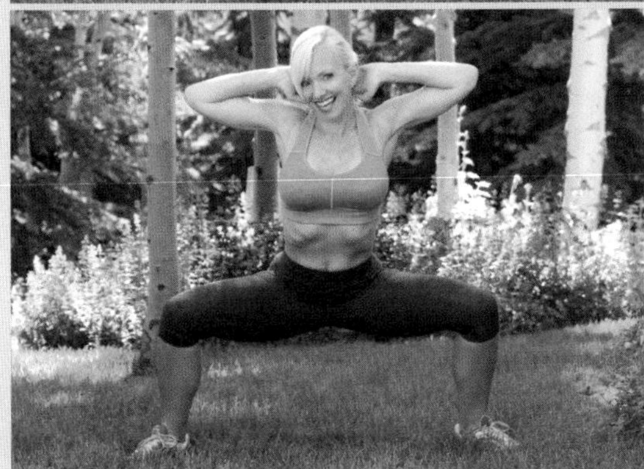

1. Put your legs together, with knees bent and arms straight down.
2. Hop and move your legs with toes pointing to corners and knees bent while your arms move to the back of your head. Stay low.
3. Repeat set 12 times, march for one minute, then repeat 12 more times. Strive to do two total sets for a total of 48.

TODAY'S LOG

EXERCISE

Description	Length of time

VEGETABLES AND FRUIT Strive for 5 servings.

1	4
2	5
3	

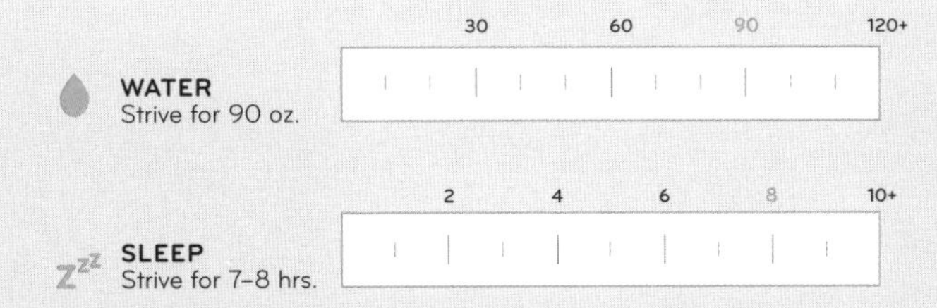

REFLECTIONS

Look back on on your progress during Week Two by recording your answers to these questions:

What healthy habit do you want to claim this week?

Since beginning this 21-Day Action Plan, in what ways are you feeling better about yourself?

What motivates you to continue making better decisions about the food you eat and the liquid you drink?

What new physical activities do you want to try in the future?

What action are you most proud of since beginning the 21-Day Action Plan?

EXERCISE SCHEDULE: Week Three

DAY 15 Interval Walk-Run for 30 minutes.
DVD OPTION: **Cardio Dance Ensemble**

DAY 16 Jog in place with high knee lifts to music for 3 minutes, 25 front push-ups and 30 back push-ups. Repeat combination three more times for a total of 100 front push-ups, 120 back push-ups and 12 minutes of high knee lift jogging.
DVD OPTION: **Full Body Strengthening**

DAY 17 Gentle walk, bike or other physical activity outdoors for 30 minutes.
No DVD option

DAY 18 Do a combination of 4 *Knock-Out Moves of the Day* of your choice.
DVD OPTION: **Cardio Dance Ensemble**

DAY 19 Jump rope for 3 minutes, 25 front push-ups and 30 back push-ups. Repeat combination three more times for a total of 100 front push-ups, 120 back push-ups and 12 minutes of jumping rope.
DVD OPTION: **Full Body Strengthening**

DAY 20 Walk briskly for 5 minutes, stop and do 25 jumping jacks followed by 15 slow squats (1,000-1 going down; 1,000-2 coming up) and 15 fast squats. Repeat three more times for a total of 100 jumping jacks, 60 slow squats, 60 fast squats and 20 minutes of brisk walking.
DVD OPTION: **Cardio Dance Ensemble**

DAY 21 Pick your four favorite *Knock-Out Moves of the Day*, turn up the music and *go fot it*!
DVD OPTION: **Full Body Strengthening**

15

"Motivation is what gets you started. Habit is what keeps you going."

JIM ROHN

Motivation and repetition are the keys to establishing healthy habits. No one can eat healthily or exercise for you. Stay motivated!

- Welcome to Week Three! Remember to weigh yourself as soon as you wake up, after going to the bathroom and before eating or drinking anything.
- Schedule your workouts and bedtimes on your calendar.
- Plan your meals and snacks for the week.
- Try on that item of clothing that is hanging as a reminder to you to stay on track. Are you seeing any improvement in the way it fits?

♥ Be a Big Brother! Be a Big Sister! Help shape a child's future for the better by empowering him/her to achieve in all areas of life. Find a local chapter near you: www.bbbs.org/site/c.9iILI3NGKh-K6F/b.5962345/k.E123/Volunteer_to_start_something.htm for more information.

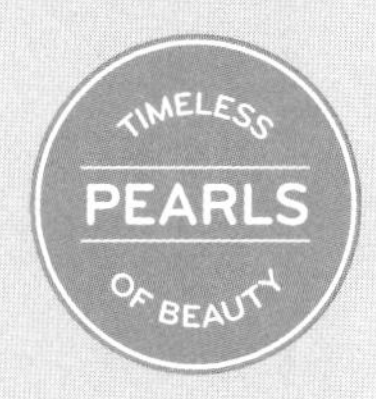

Stay personally connected with friends by phoning or having FaceTime. Talking with someone who loves you is very uplifting, even if it's only for a few precious minutes.

KNOCK-OUT MOVE OF THE DAY

SQUAT PULSE

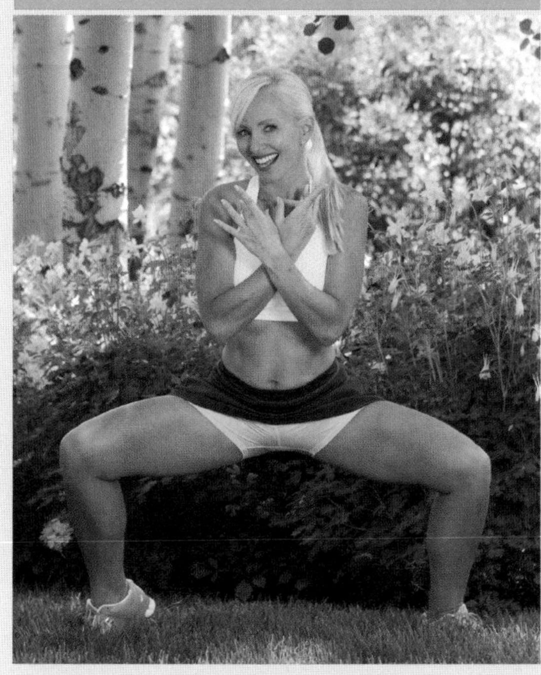

1. Stand in the "V" position with toes pointed to corners, knees bent and arms across your chest.
2. With one toe popped and your heel up, pulse up and down (staying low) 24 times then switch legs.
3. Repeat two times for a total of 48 pulses on each leg.

TODAY'S LOG

CURRENT WEIGHT

EXERCISE

Description	Length of time

VEGETABLES AND FRUIT Strive for 5 servings.

1	4
2	5
3	

WATER
Strive for 90 oz.

30 60 90 120+

SLEEP
Strive for 7–8 hrs.

2 4 6 8 10+

16

"Health is a state of complete harmony of the body, mind and spirit. When one is free from physical disabilities and mental distractions, the gates of the soul open." "

B.K.S. IYENGAR

As you get active, it's common for insecurities to surface, for you to recall times you felt shame or embarrassment about your body, your coordination or your risk taking. Let the feelings rise, and love yourself through any anguish or tears. Then set the feelings aside and affirm yourself for the great new habits you are forming. Feel beautiful and strong, just the way you are.

- Take good care of yourself. We are often so busy caring for family, friends and others in our community that we forget about ourselves. But a stronger *"you"* can fend off illness and create the energy and inspiration you need to take advantage of all that life has to offer.
- Fill up a bowl with ice water then dunk your face in and out of it for one minute. This activity brings out the color in your cheeks, tightens your face and wakes you up.
- To soothe a burn from all the cooking you're doing, rub raw honey on the spot. The sugary nectar may speed healing time by as much as four days.
- ♥ Clean out your closet and donate shoes, purses, suits, shirts, pants and coats to a local shelter that offers professional clothing to needy women and men.

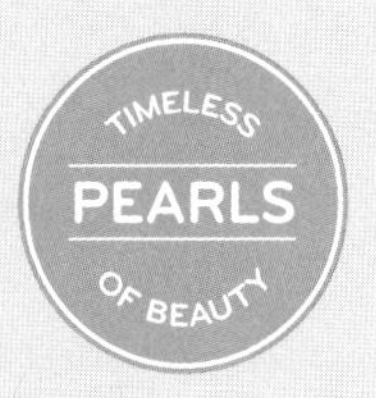

Moisturize before bed, applying Aquaphor® to your chest, the tops of your hands, and heels of your feet. You'll slow down the signs of aging.

KNOCK-OUT MOVE OF THE DAY

SIDE LIFT

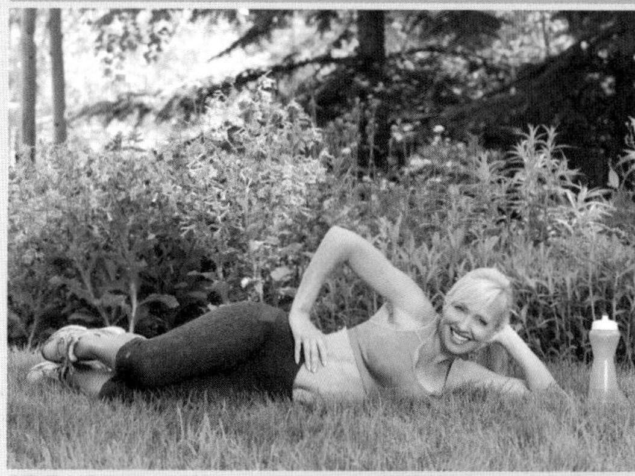

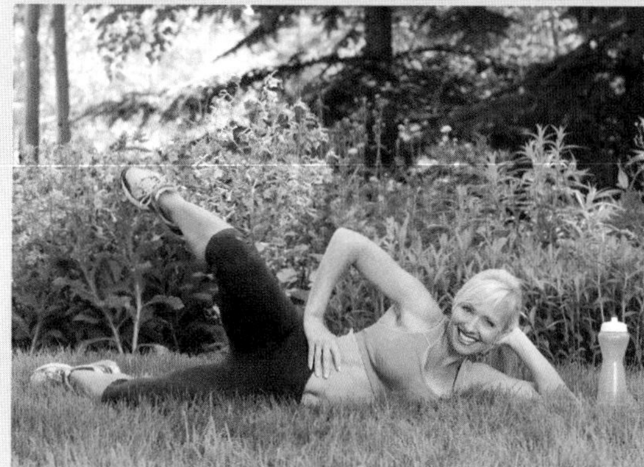

1. Lying on your side with legs slightly bent and toes pointed, raise your top leg and keep it parallel to your bottom leg.
2. Lower the leg and repeat 24 times then switch sides so that the opposite top leg does the lift.

TODAY'S LOG

EXERCISE

Description	Length of time

VEGETABLES AND FRUIT Strive for 5 servings.

1	4
2	5
3	

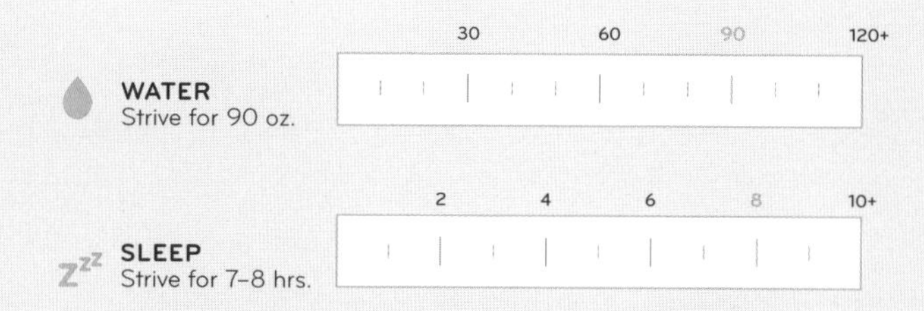

17 "Truly *live* your life and experience how it will love you in return."

MOLLY SHATTUCK

Take advantage of every minute — this is your life. Do something you enjoy every day. It's these little moments of happiness that improve the quality of your life. We don't get back yesterday or last year.

- Set high, yet achievable personal goals, and rejoice when you reach them. Those who do this are "more satisfied" in life, according to Tal Ben-Shahar, Ph.D., and author of *The Pursuit of Perfect*.
- Keep repeating your healthy actions each day and they soon will turn into habits that can be sustained for life.
- Wrap your arms around yourself for two minutes. And give six-second hugs to others.
- Take 21 minutes today to close your eyes and focus on slow and peaceful breathing. Allow yourself to fully relax. Warning: You may want to set an alarm before you try this.

♥ Connect with people around the world to help alleviate poverty by lending $25, following the small business you help create, getting your investment back and lending it to another person's efforts. To learn more, visit www.kiva.org.

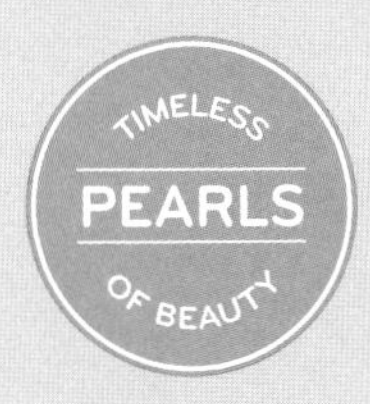

Add celery to your smoothies and snacks to naturally tighten your skin. For more cellulose power, pop cold cucumber slices on your eyelids for 15 minutes and walk away looking bright-eyed and cheery!

KNOCK-OUT MOVE OF THE DAY

SIDE EXTEND LIFT

1. Lying on your side with the lower leg bent and toes pointed, lift the top leg, keeping it parallel to the bottom leg, then lower back down.
2. Repeat 24 times then switch legs so that the opposite leg lifts.

TODAY'S LOG

EXERCISE

Description	Length of time

VEGETABLES AND FRUIT Strive for 5 servings.

1	4
2	5
3	

WATER
Strive for 90 oz.

30 60 90 120+

SLEEP
Strive for 7–8 hrs.

2 4 6 8 10+

18

"Every healthy decision you make matters."

MOLLY SHATTUCK

Choosing water over soda, vegetables over chips and a brisk walk over the urge to attack the cookie jar? These choices all add up to a healthier you. It's our daily, small decisions that make *all the difference* when it comes to creating positive habits that can be sustained throughout our lives.

- Chew out calories. Chew a fork/spoonful of food 20 or more times for every bite you take. There's a good chance you'll become full more quickly and reduce your calorie intake by a meaningful amount. And remember to drink 12 gulps of water before each meal.
- Begin working on your new or revived hobby and inspire others in the Vibrant Living Community at www.mollyshattuck.com.
- Make time to begin thinking about the goals you want to set for yourself this year and beyond. Start making plans to achieve them.
- Avoid mindless eating and savor every bite. Don't eat in front of the T.V. or computer. Focus on your eating, and you'll probably be satisfied with a smaller amount of food.
- Make dinner an event this weekend. Set the table carefully with your best dishes or some cheerful paper plates. Play soothing music in the background, and create an elegant mood by putting fresh flowers on the table and eating by candlelight.

♥ Host a healthy food drive at your school or business. Visit www.mollyshattuck.com to learn how.

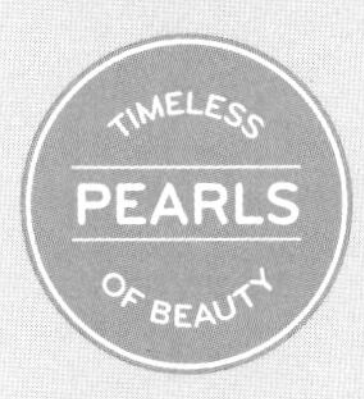

Floss daily to strengthen your immune system. Bacteria in the mouth can travel directly to the heart. If our bodies are in a constant state of fighting bacteria, we weaken our energy supply.

KNOCK-OUT MOVE OF THE DAY

CROSS INNER LIFT

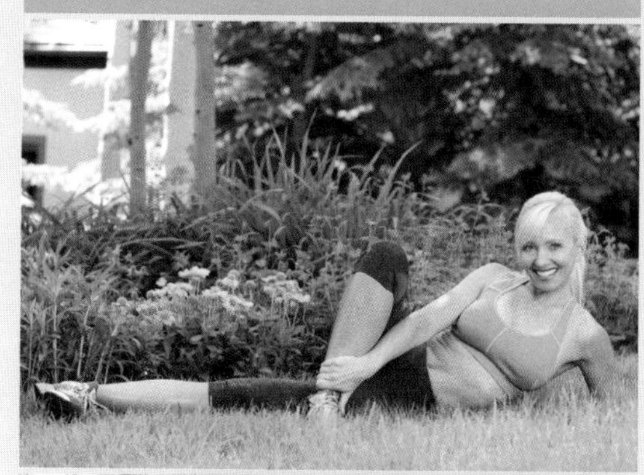

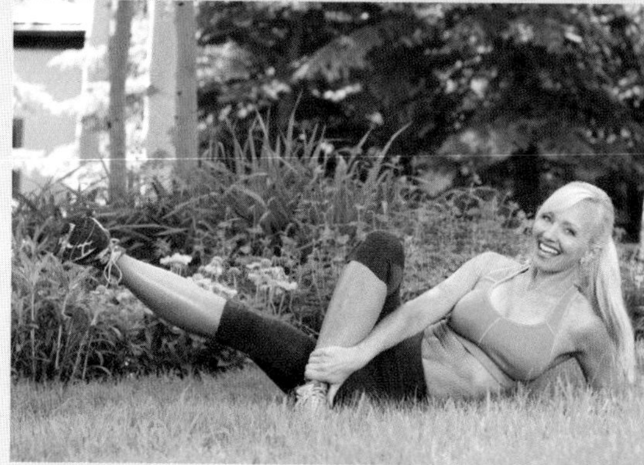

1. Lie on your side with the bottom lower leg straight and the foot flexed. Cross your top leg over the bottom leg.
2. Raise the bottom leg and lower it to ground, keeping parallel with the sky.
3. Repeat it 24 times and switch sides so that the opposite leg does the lift.

TODAY'S LOG

EXERCISE

Description	Length of time

VEGETABLES AND FRUIT Strive for 5 servings.

1	4
2	5
3	

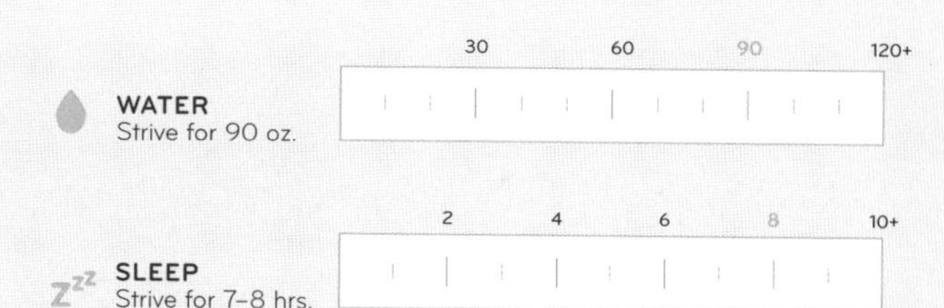

19 "The meaning of life is in the details."

MOLLY SHATTUCK

The fine details of any event or moment make it sparkle. Why wait for an "occasion" to add glitz to your life? Do it today!

- Stay focused. The more committed to improving your health you become, the better your chances of avoiding health-related complications in the future.
- Play beautiful, calming music while you cook.
- Be aware of your coworkers' and friends' eating and drinking habits, as they may be influencing your choices. A recent study at the University of Cincinnati found that people who are together on a regular basis often adopt each other's eating styles and habits, especially when it comes to snacking and alcohol consumption. To keep others' bad habits at bay, fill up on healthy food choices like fruits and vegetables. Limit late-night eating, and encourage your acquaintances to get healthier *with* you. Let your good habits rub off on them.

♥ Support your neighborhood kids at a local YMCA, bolstering youth development, healthy living and social responsibility initiatives. For more information, visit www.ymca.net/volunteer.

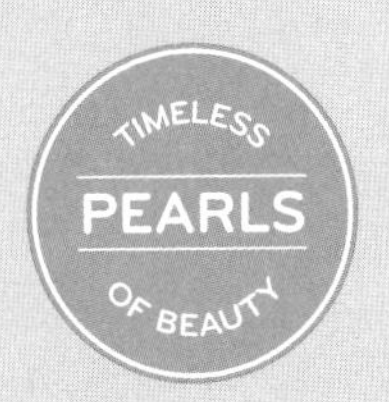

Exfoliate and cleanse your face every day. Daily Resurfacing Disks® by ROC significantly improve the skin's appearance.

KNOCK-OUT MOVE OF THE DAY

SWITCH ARMS

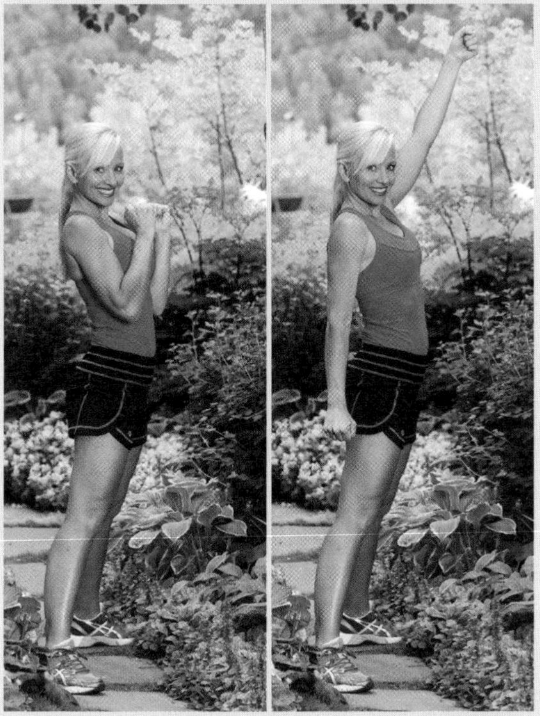

1. Start by standing with your legs apart, shoulders back. Point your toes to the corners with your arms bent and fists facing each other.
2. Raise one arm straight up and, at the same time, lower the other arm.
3. Alternate your arms 24 times, up and down. Do a total of 48—or more if the music hasn't stopped or the commercial hasn't ended.

TODAY'S LOG

EXERCISE

Description	Length of time

VEGETABLES AND FRUIT Strive for 5 servings.

1	4
2	5
3	

WATER
Strive for 90 oz.

30 60 90 120+

SLEEP
Strive for 7–8 hrs.

2 4 6 8 10+

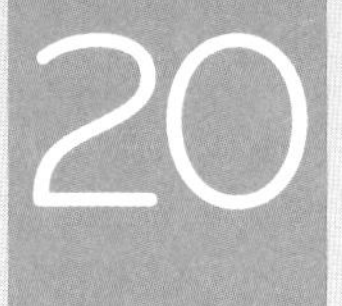

"Every challenge has a limited lifespan when you choose to do something about it." "

MOLLY SHATTUCK

You are in charge of your life. Don't allow yourself to be held down by challenges; simply find ways to work through them. You are a beautiful, smart person who has great potential to do and get exactly what you want in life. Go create the opportunities and let every decision you make support your ultimate goals.

- Create colorful meals and make them look pretty on the plate.
- Encourage each person you know to drink more water, eat more fresh vegetables and fruit, exercise daily and help other people when possible. You could be the one to save another's life.
- Schedule an extra walk with someone you love this week.
- Rethink your role model. Find someone who is REAL and alive today. Look for a person who is friendly, strong, kind and likes animals and kids.
- Forgive yourself for when you make mistakes and forgive others for doing the same. And be the first to apologize.

♥ Give the gift of groceries to our military service members through Commissary Gift Certificates at www.commissaries.com/giftcard.

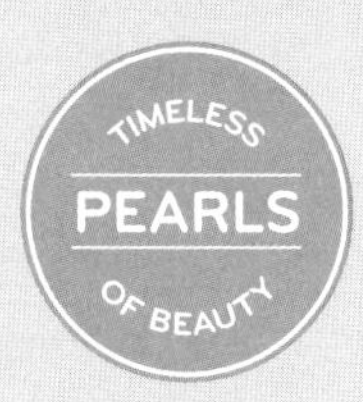

Inhale deeply through your nose and exhale through your mouth to regain control — in exercise and in tense moments. Let your shoulders drop!

KNOCK-OUT MOVE OF THE DAY

EXTENSION LIFTS

1. Get on both hands, with one knee bent and the other straight, chin up.
2. Lift the extended leg up with toes pointed. Lower it back to the ground.
3. Repeat 24 times and switch legs so the opposite leg does the lift.

TODAY'S LOG

EXERCISE

Description	Length of time

VEGETABLES AND FRUIT Strive for 5 servings.

1
2
3
4
5

	30	60	90	120+
WATER Strive for 90 oz.				

	2	4	6	8	10+
SLEEP Strive for 7–8 hrs.					

21

"Don't look for God in the sky;
look within your own body." "

OSHO

All elements of your life are connected. You honor God by honoring your body and the earth. You are built to serve, and now have energy to live your life with higher purpose.

- Make every day matter. Infuse your life with quality; your happiness and vitality depends on it.
- Live your life with a healthy twist, no matter what you're doing.
- Today is the first day—to start incorporating all of the 21-Day Action Plan lessons you've learned into the rest of your life!
- Remember why you embarked on the 21-Day Action Plan. Transformation happens when you intentionally put effort into it each and every day.
- Find humor in your life every day.
  "I don't understand sizes anymore. There's a size zero which I didn't even know they had. It must stand for 'Ooooh, my God, you're thin.'" — Ellen DeGeneres

♥ Get together with friends and make homemade cookies. Deliver them to an elder care facility in your neighborhood or town.

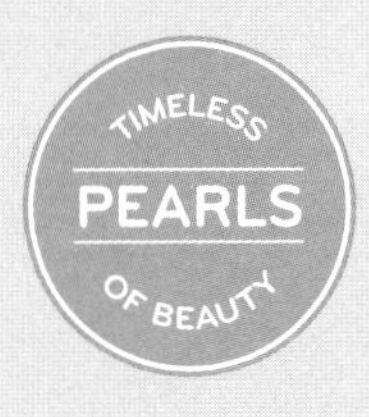

Read an inspiring thought every day. Print your favorites and hang them on your mirror, refrigerator or keep a few on your bedside table.

KNOCK-OUT MOVE OF THE DAY

REV UP

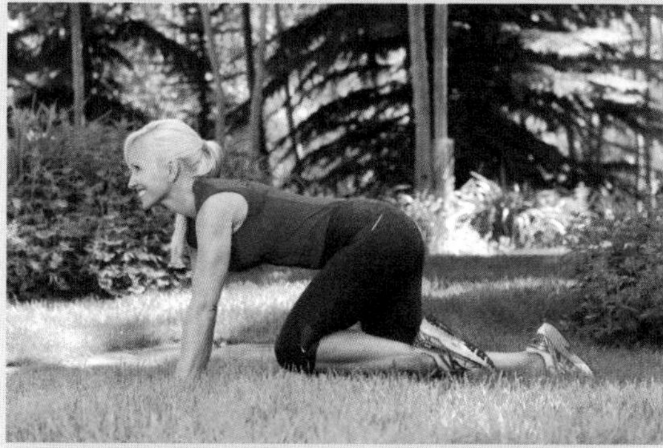

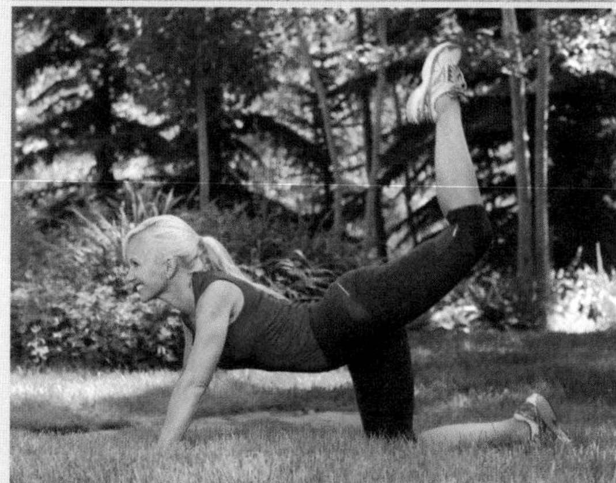

1. Get on all fours with your arms straight, chin up and the left leg slightly forward.
2. Lift and extend the left leg back and up, while pointing your toes. Lower it to the ground.
3. Repeat 24 times and change up so the opposite leg goes up and down.

TODAY'S LOG

EXERCISE

Description	Length of time

VEGETABLES AND FRUIT Strive for 5 servings.

1	4
2	5
3	

WATER
Strive for 90 oz.

30 60 90 120+

SLEEP
Strive for 7–8 hrs.

2 4 6 8 10+

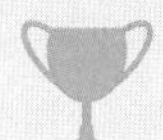

WELL DONE!
You have completed the 21-Day Action Plan!
Turn the page to record your results.

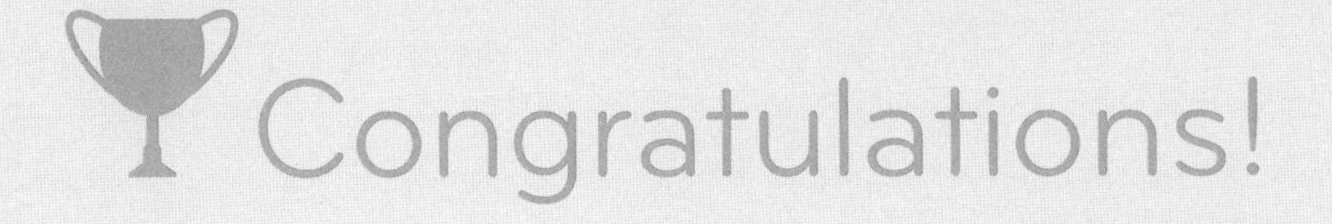

Congratulations!

For the past 21 days you have taken positive steps to improve your health. That's a great accomplishment.

RESULTS OF YOUR 21-DAY ACTION PLAN

Now's the time to see how much your body is changing and how well your habits are forming. Take stock and then take action—so that you continue to reap rewards of Molly Vibrant Living.

Current weight:

Inches melted away:

Pounds lost:

Average daily average ounces of water consumed:

Average hours of sleep each night:

Number of days you exercised each week:

What's next for you?
Read on to get some ideas . . .

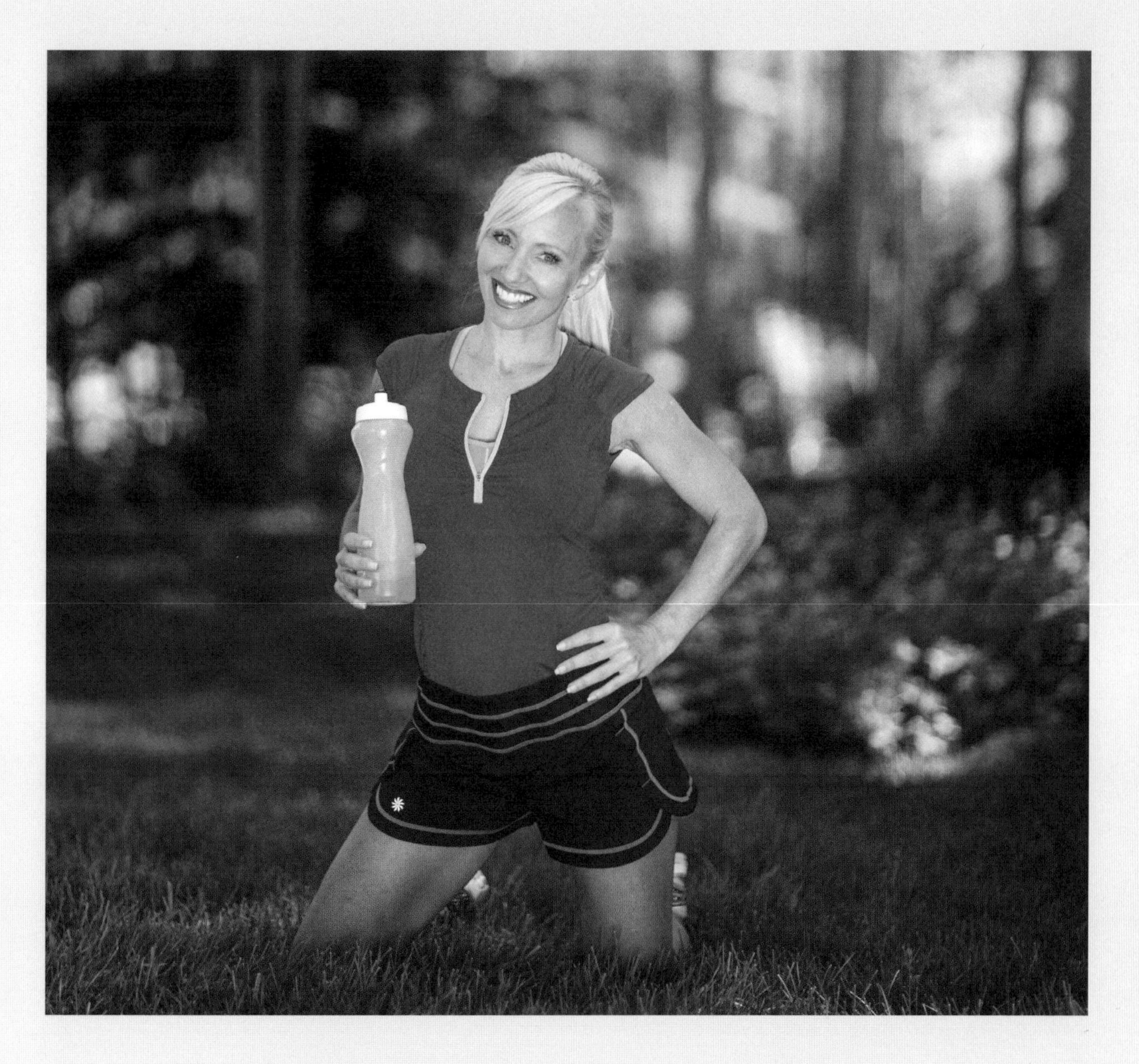

Beyond 21 Days

CREATING A ROADMAP FOR THE REST OF YOUR LIFE

"Understand that the right to choose your own path is a sacred privilege. Use it. Dwell in possibility."
—*Oprah Winfrey*

Congratulations! For the past 21 days, you've honored your body, taking meaningful and positive steps to improve your health. You've incorporated some new habits—increasing your water intake, eating more REAL food, exercising more frequently and living for others. I do hope that you are now experiencing the perks—higher energy, weight loss, reduced headaches, healthier looking skin, increased muscle tone, better moods, increased libido and a feeling of greater passion and purpose in your life.

Along the way, you probably found that changing a behavior can be tough. A disciplined approach to healthier practices in your life is *hard work*. But without this deliberate action, nothing was going to change about the way you looked or the way you felt—except that with age, it might have gotten a bit worse. So *feel proud of your accomplishments*. Your consciousness about everyday habits will dramatically change the way you look and feel in the weeks, months and years to come.

How can you ensure that your new habits become ingrained and long lasting? When tomorrow's big opportunity comes, as I suggested in the beginning of the book, will you have the health and energy to enable you to snap it up?

I'm confident you won't revert to your old self, and even if you do slip up a bit, you can look back at your daily log, breathe in some of the motivation you felt, forgive yourself and start again. Look upon these weeks as your training camp. You learned the fundamentals and practiced them over and over until they started to become second nature. And now you're ready to start living your life in a more dynamic, intentional way. Feeling good about your physical self can give you the confidence to achieve any ambitions and desires you have.

So . . . what do you want to do *next*?

ONE DECISION CAN CHANGE EVERYTHING

About a year before I graduated from high school, my mom and I began planning a trek to the bottom of the Grand Canyon. We were careful, as we scheduled our trip, taking into consideration both the weather conditions in the canyon and the milestone moments of my senior year. But, at the last minute, my high school changed the date of my senior prom and it ended up being scheduled at the same time as our mother-daughter trip to Arizona.

Like most teenage girls, I had long looked forward to my high school prom—and one of the first opportunities I had to dress "like a grown-up." My friends and I spent hours shopping for the perfect dresses, practicing our make-up, and poring over fashion magazines for the right hairstyles. Yet, after agonizing over the dilemma—between the prom and the trip—I decided to hike the Grand Canyon with my mom.

Hiking the Grand Canyon was an extraordinary three-day experience. We hiked through a wind storm, rain, snow and blistering heat, and saw awe-inspiring vistas at every turn. On the night we arrived at the base of the canyon, my mom and I sat around a campfire, two adventurers looking up at the limitless sky of dazzling stars.

Something inside of me ignited. The awesomeness of nature was spread out before me. The possibility of being an entrepreneur, a mother and an adventurer was born in me. That's when I decided to live my life *on my terms*. I would determine what I wanted and figure out how to get it, rather than sitting on the sidelines and waiting for life to happen to me.

I pulled out a notebook I was carrying in my backpack and made a list of 10 personal goals. This list turned out to be the roadmap for my life. Some items were commonly held desires, such as getting married and having a family. But others, including getting a college degree, climbing Mount Kilimanjaro, becoming an NFL cheerleader and a Rockette, were pretty big dreams for a senior in high school from a very small town in Pennsylvania.

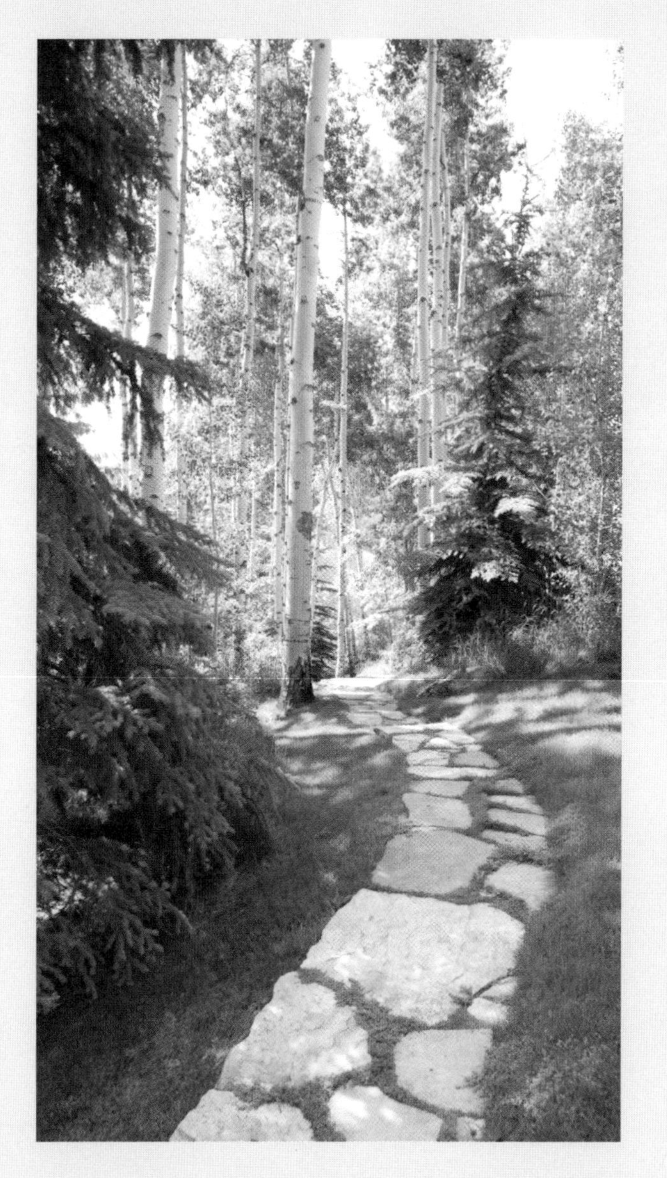

Yet, from the moment I put those goals in writing, I began to make daily choices that would get me closer to reaching them. I've now achieved most of the goals on that original list. The 5'7" height limit has made me ineligible to audition for the Rockettes. But I'm still hoping they'll change the requirement—or perhaps I'll grow taller. There's also that little matter of my being older than their age limit now, but there's always a chance they'll extend it!

The decision to go to the Grand Canyon didn't just change my life, it *created* the *direction* of my life. Each day sincerely matters, and so does every decision you make. Setting goals, looking for the good in every situation, moving forward with confidence instead of being stuck in the past—all of these are vibrant and intentional approaches to life.

CREATING *YOUR* ROADMAP FOR LIFE

I started my list 28 years ago—the list of 10 goals I dreamed of accomplishing in my lifetime. That list now has approximately 50 items on it, many of which are checked off while some are in the planning stages and many others await attention.

This year I returned to the Canyon to do the hike I did many years ago. This time, however, I did the 21.5 miles of it with 12,000 feet of elevation change, all in a single day. My experience was different than when I had my original epiphany; it was a grounding experience of sorts. I realized I've found my sweet spot in life, doing what I love: being a mom, a volunteer and a community leader, while helping others get healthy. During the trip, I made it my mission to finish this book so that I could help more people.

Now that you're in better control of your personal health, it's time to start taking charge of your future. The first step is to begin designing your own *Roadmap for Life*.

Think about what you really want out of life, based on your values, interests and priorities. What inspires and excites you? The act of writing down a goal on paper is the first step in turning dreams into plans of action. The saying "out of sight, out of mind" holds true with dreams. If you don't have them written down staring you in the face, you're less likely to ever pursue them and have regrets later in life. So . . .

1. Identify the steps you need to take along the way to reach your goals and commit to them. Remember, no goal is too big or too small—simply own it!
2. Establish mini goals and major goals on an ongoing basis—and write them down! That way, you will be motivated to work harder to make them happen.
3. Create measurable and specific goals to which you can attach a date, time frame or some other significant marker. Writing down that you want to "lose weight" has much less impact than writing about your desire to "lose 10 pounds by Christmas day by eliminating junk food and eating five servings of vegetables and fruit each day."

This goal-writing exercise can be the beginning of your list of life goals. It's the first step of your *Roadmap for Life*, which you will refine as your interests and priorities shift.

To help you get started, below are some areas one which you may want to focus to give structure to your *Roadmap*.

This year I want to begin to:

This year I want to finish:

Health goals:

Places I want to visit:

Skills or hobbies I want to develop:

Experiences I want to have:

Fears I want to overcome:

Ways I can strengthen relationships:

ONE LAST PEP TALK

It's time to use the skills you've learned—and the vibrant energy you've developed—to pursue your goals and infuse your life with as much joy and fulfillment as you possibly can. But first, let me give you one last pep talk.

As you've worked through this book, I hope you have come to realize that *you* are in control of your life, starting with how you choose to view yourself and the world around you. You decide how every situation, pitfall and victory will impact you. You can turn setbacks and mistakes into learning opportunities, and make your positive attitude the graceful and fluid paintbrush of your life portrait.

Focus on the "good" in each day and acknowledge even your smallest achievements. In my evening bath before bed, I often feel a sense of closure and take great satisfaction in knowing my kitchen is clean, the laundry is folded and my kids are snuggled in their beds. I've checked off "to-do" list items and started a new list for the next day. Everything you accomplish deserves recognition. I urge you to applaud your small, daily joys and cherish the rituals that help you feel settled and at peace.

Learn to persevere by watching and celebrating the journeys of others around you, people who encounter unexpected bumps in the road but go on to turn detours into sacred destinations. In my experience, fear and procrastination are great teachers. If you're avoiding getting something done, *do it first*. Eat your fear—*before* breakfast! Do the hard task, and then rejoice at the fact that you did it. Each time you conquer a fear, each time you vanquish an anxiety, you will think of yourself as a conquerer and a survivor. You will carry yourself with more confidence, living more joyfully, by denying fear and doubt from having power over your life. *Don't ask God to make your life easier. Ask God to make you a stronger person.*

Say grace. Be thankful. Incorporate habits—drinking water, eating real food, exercising daily and living for others—so that your body is a vessel for grace, compassion and strength.

Create a virtuous circle of support, calling on members of the Molly Vibrant Living community and people who fuel, not deplete, your energy.

Pause. Think. Act. Live your life on your terms. Walk away from the things that limit you and rely on God as your source of strength and sustenance.

Cultivate opportunities to find deeper meaning in life. Go after what you know is right for you, listening to and trusting your inner voice. Turn your routines into treasured rituals. Let your passion drive you, as you take ownership of your life, your daily choices and your future, regardless of what others might think. Respond to God, and to the many gifts you have been given, with vibrant energy.

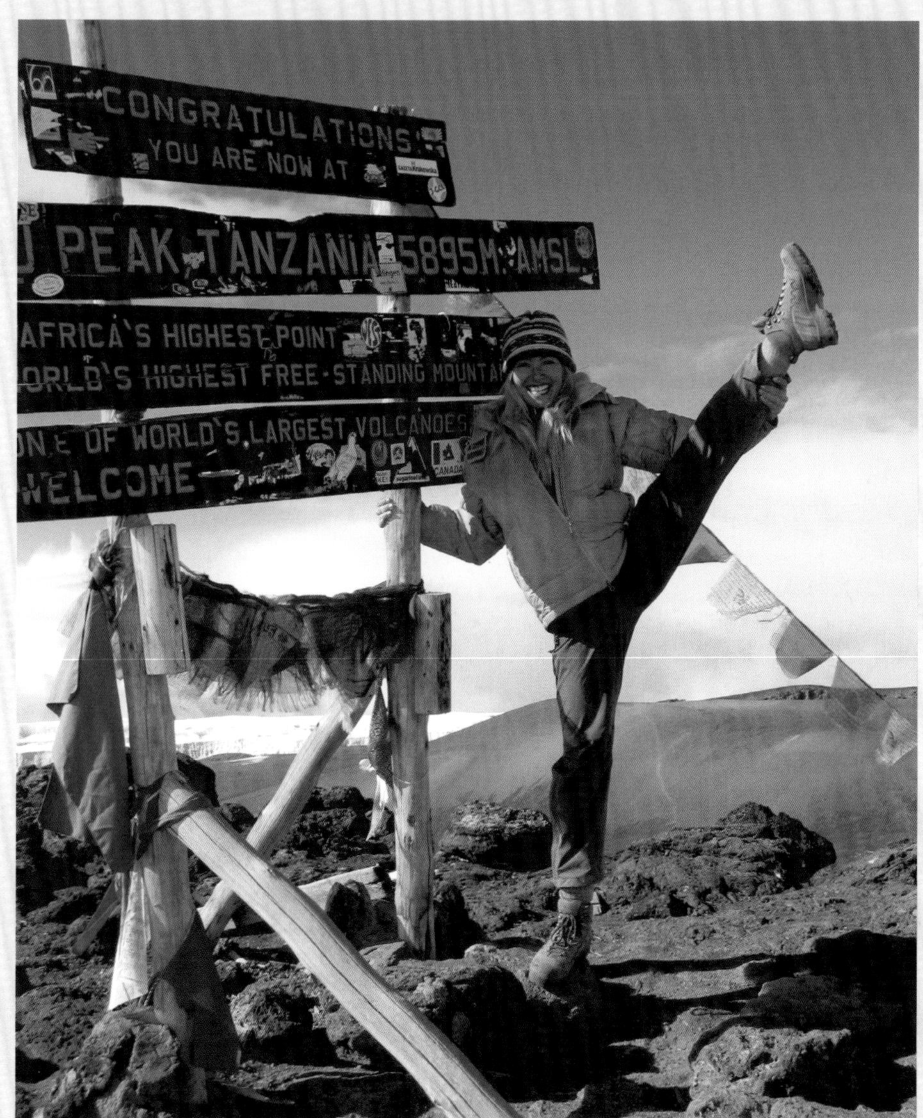

Summit of Mount Kilimanjaro, October 2007.

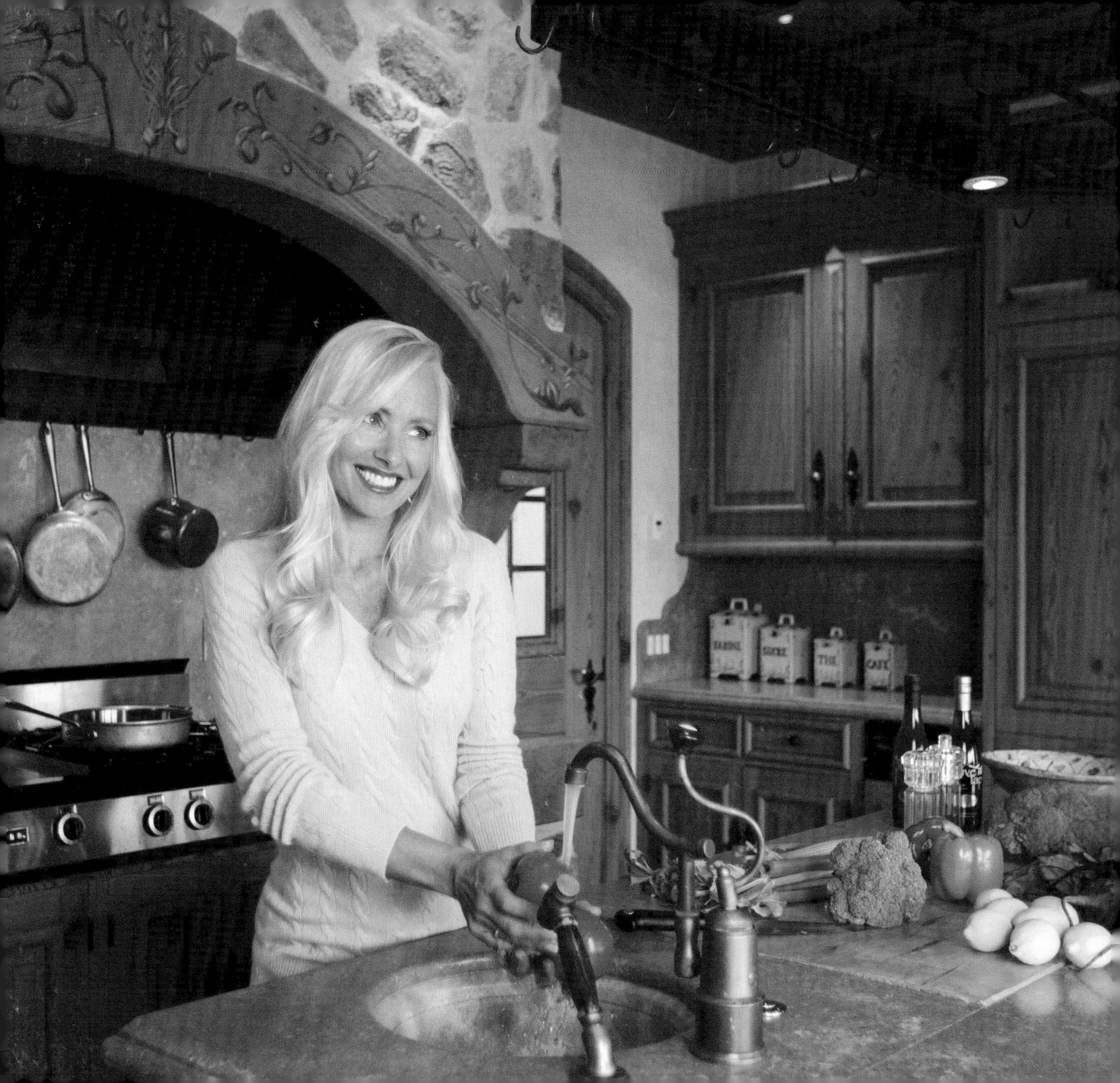

MAKE *REAL* MEALS

You can do this! Enjoy these easy-to-make meals and snacks. They're for busy people who want to take control of their health with fresh ingredients and scrumptious food.

Simple REAL Meals

Be in total control of the food you put in your body. Prepare the majority of your meals in your own kitchen and take food with you when possible. Cooking your own meals is one of the best ways to take charge of what you eat. It also helps ensure you consume more vegetables, fiber, legumes, whole grains and lean meats, and that you limit the amount of "bad" fat, salt and sugar in your food. And, as a bonus, you will save a lot of money.

The suggestions on the following pages for breakfast, lunch, dinner, snacks and dessert are part of my personal history. Some of the recipes have been passed on in my family for generations and others are newly discovered from magazines and cookbooks. The recipes I've selected have three things in common: they are delicious, nutritious and easy to prepare.

I enjoy trying new combinations of foods and learning more about how to better care for my family, my community and myself. I have discovered that cooking with friends, family, fellow church members and total strangers creates an instant sense of community. There is something cozy and rewarding about connecting with others over food, and it's vital to a healthy lifestyle.

A few general points to keep in mind: Be sure to always rinse fruits, vegetables, fish and meat as a first step in preparation. Wash lids on cans before opening them and rinse the contents of single-ingredient canned goods such as peas, corn or beans to wash away salt and preservatives. When fresh or frozen vegetables are not options, choose low- or no-sodium canned varieties. And control your fat intake by using a spray bottle with extra virgin olive oil to prepare pans and dress food.

Get creative and experiment with different combinations to pump up the nutritional value of your meals. Below is a list of some healthy substitutions for commonly used ingredients you might want to consider:

- Unsweetened applesauce for sugar
- Avocado puree for butter
- Cacao nibs for chocolate chips
- Shredded zucchini or spaghetti squash for pasta
- Mashed turnips or cauliflower for mashed potatoes
- Rolled oats for bread crumbs
- Arugula, romaine, spinach and kale for iceberg lettuce
- Baked kale chips for potato chips
- Low-fat mayonnaise or sour cream for vegetable oil

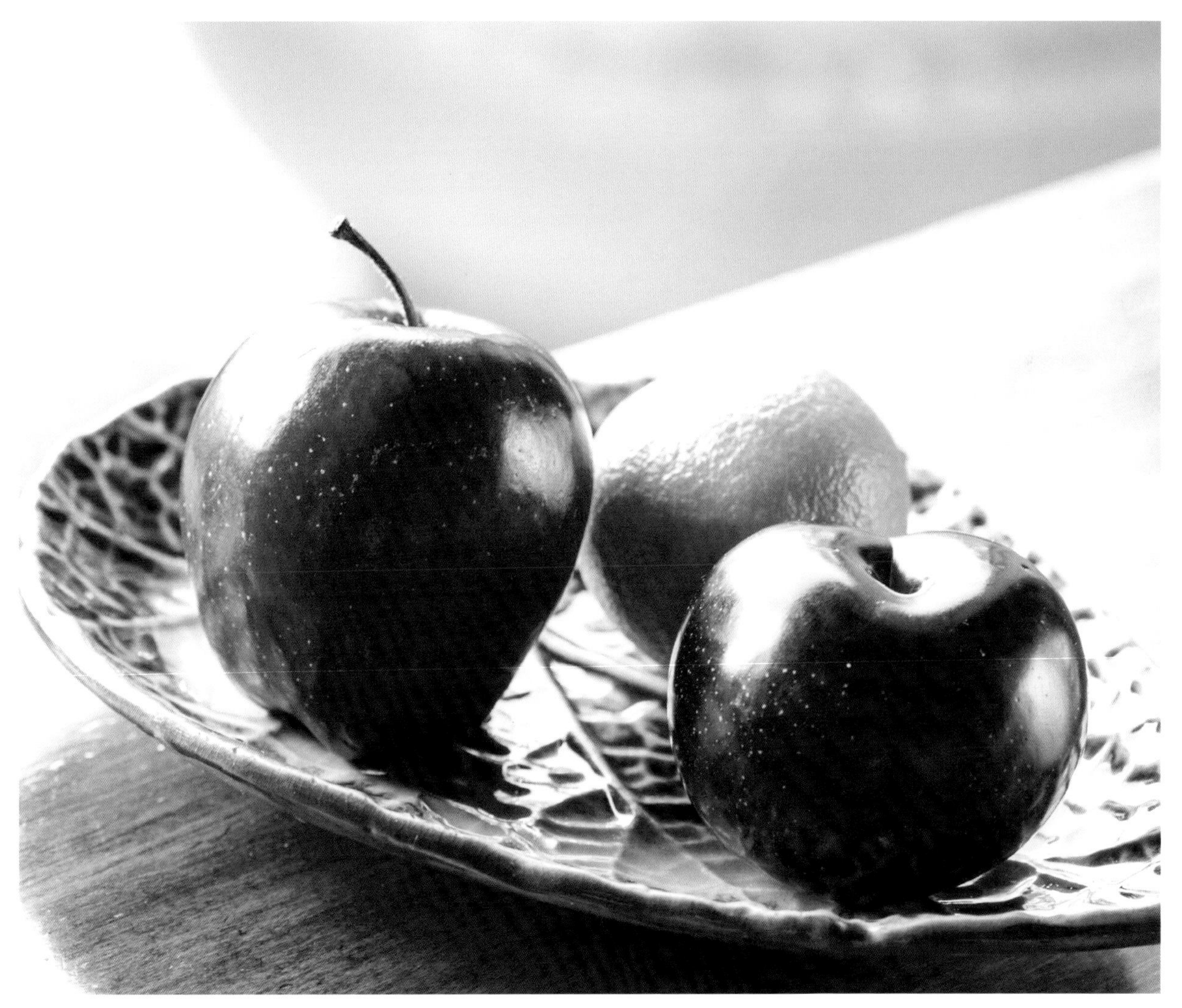

Rinse fruits and veggies thoroughly. Wash away salt and preservatives on canned items, too.

Rise and Shine with Breakfast

After drinking 30 ounces of water to begin your day, always eat fruit first, choosing items from the *Grocery List* (page 82), such as half of a pink or red grapefruit, an apple with skin, one cup of mixed berries or half a banana.

Plus, choose from the following:

- ½ cup All Bran® plus ¾ cup Special K® or other whole grain cereals that have fiber, fewer than 6 grams of sugar, fewer than 2 grams of fat and less than 10% sodium (daily value per serving). Top with one-half cup of 1% milk.
- Plain Greek yogurt with fresh berries and/or ½ cup Fiber One®, Special K®, Cheerios® or Total® cereal.
- Rolled oats with 1% milk and sprinkled with cinnamon or 1 Tbsp. dark brown sugar. Avoid artificial sweeteners! If you choose to add sugar, be in charge of the amount you consume and stay away from flavored oatmeal packets.
- One whole wheat, multi-grain, multi-grain fiber, triple health or health-full English muffin or one slice of whole grain toast with either 1 Tbsp. Simply Jif® peanut butter or 1 tsp. unsalted butter, with or without jelly.
- 1 or 2 hard-boiled* or scrambled egg(s). Use extra virgin olive oil or a tsp. of unsalted butter with a light sprinkle of cheese and chunks of tomato with any fresh vegetables.
- Fresh fruit smoothie made with large handful of spinach or kale. Use any combination of 1 cup berries, kiwi, ½ peeled apple cut into chunks, ½ banana, ½ cup pineapple and any other fruit you desire. Add a handful of ice, five unsalted almonds and 2 Tbsp. 100% orange juice or 2 Tbsp. yogurt of your choice. Mix well in a blender.

* Directions for hard boiled eggs: Remove eggs from refrigerator and let stand to reach room temperature. Fill large pot with water, cover and place pot over high heat. Once water is boiling, carefully place eggs in pot and cook for 12 minutes. Rinse eggs in cool water and peel. Serving size is 1 egg. Combine this with fresh vegetables and you will be satisfied and full of energy!

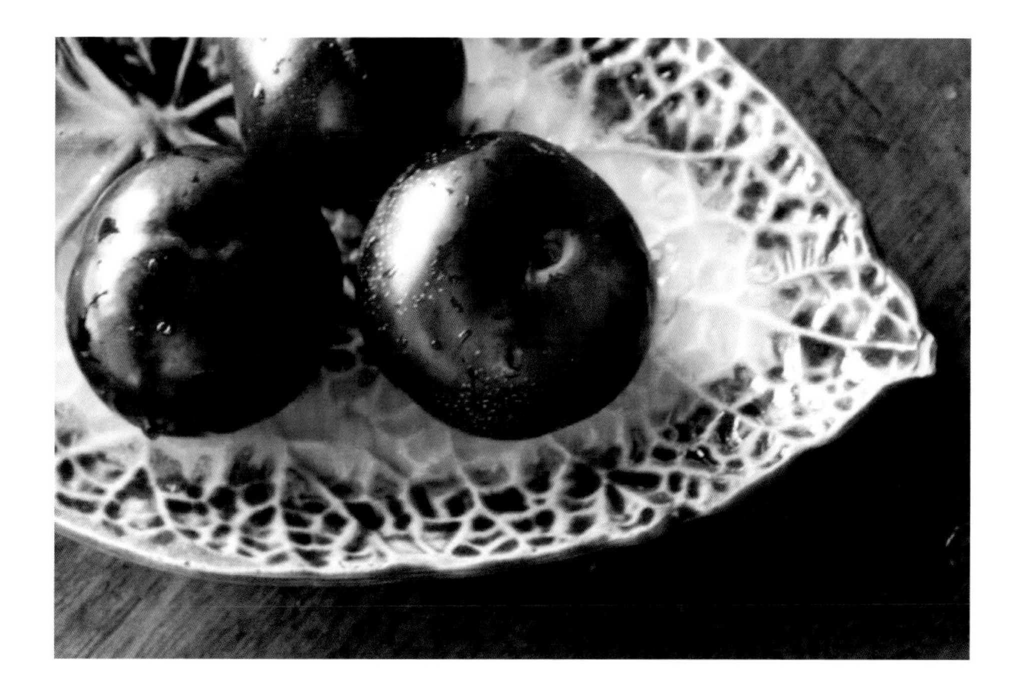

BERRY BRAN MUFFINS

Ingredients for 12 muffins:
1 ½ cups wheat bran
1 cup 1% milk
½ cup unsweetened applesauce
1 egg
⅔ cup brown sugar
½ tsp. lemon extract
1 tsp. lemon rind
½ cup all-purpose unbleached flour
½ cup whole wheat flour
1 tsp. baking powder
1 tsp. baking soda
1 cup blueberries or raspberries, rinsed well

Directions: Preheat oven to 350°. Line 12-cup muffin tin with paper liners. Mix together wheat bran and milk, and let stand for 10 minutes. In a large bowl, mix together applesauce, egg, brown sugar, and vanilla. Beat in bran mixture. Sift together all-purpose flour, whole wheat flour, baking soda and baking powder. Stir into bran mixture until just blended. Fold in berries. Scoop into muffin cups with ice-cream scoop. Bake in preheated oven for 15 to 20 minutes, or until tops spring back when lightly tapped.

Homemade Take-Out Lunches

Once you've stocked up on the healthy staples on the *Grocery List* (page 82), you can throw together some quick, nourishing and delicious lunches that will keep you satisfied and energized throughout the afternoon.

Here are some of my favorites.

- Egg, spinach, cheese and avocado. Whisk together 1 egg with a splash of milk in a cereal bowl sprayed with extra virgin olive oil and bake in microwave for 45 seconds. Sprinkle a few small chunks of cheese on top and cook 10 more seconds. Serve over bed of fresh spinach with a few chunks of avocado and any other veggies.
- Salad of mixed greens with any kind of vegetables, raw or steamed. Add grilled chicken or salmon (no salt or sauce) for protein. 2 Tbsp. cheese is fine, with dressing (olive oil and vinegar is best) on the side. Dip fork in dressing instead of pouring the dressing on the salad. See *Molly's Vinaigrette* recipes (page 172).
- Open-faced sandwich with roasted turkey breast, a few chunks of cheese, tomato, cucumbers, spinach, lettuce and a side of vegetables from the *Grocery List* (page 82). Use 1 Tbsp. of light mayonnaise or Dijon mustard. If you want chips, have 1 serving. Choose those made with "real" ingredients (sliced potatoes with olive, sunflower or safflower oil should be the first ingredients on the label) and free of artificial additives and preservatives. I like Kettle Brand Bakes® or Simply 7™ Lentil Chips.

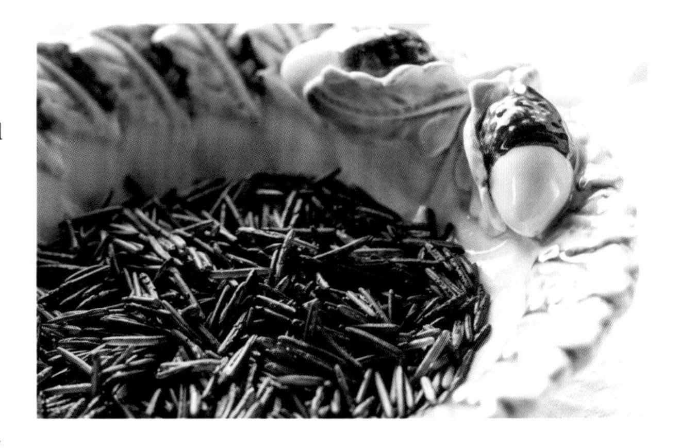

- ½ baked potato, skin on, with steamed vegetables, fresh leafy greens and one Tbsp. of cheese.

MOLLY'S CHOP CHOP SALAD

Ingredients for 4 servings:

1 bunch Romaine lettuce, rinsed well and chopped into bite-size chunks
1 bunch spinach, rinsed well and chopped into bite-size chunks
1 15.5 oz. can chick peas, rinsed and drained
1 15 oz. can black beans, rinsed and drained
2 tomatoes, rinsed well and chopped into bite-size chunks
1 cucumber with skin, rinsed well and chopped into bite-size chunks
1 avocado, rinsed well, cut in half, removed from skin and chopped into bite-size chunks
1 boneless and skinless chicken breast boiled about 20 minutes and chopped into bite-size chunks
¾ cup feta cheese

Directions: Combine all ingredients in large bowl with soft spatula. Add 3 Tbsp. of one of the *Olive Oil Vinaigrettes* on page 172.

BROWN RICE BOWL

Ingredients for 1 serving:

1 cup brown rice, cooked
2 cups fresh spinach
¾ cup roasted turkey or chicken breast, shredded or in chunks
1 Tbsp. Parmesan cheese
1 Tbsp. olive oil combined with ¼ tsp. red wine vinegar *or* 1 Tbsp. low-sodium teriyaki sauce

Directions: Place cooked rice in bowl and toss together with spinach, meat, and cheese. Drizzle dressing on top.

TUNA-EGG SALAD

Ingredients for 2 servings:

1 can albacore white tuna in water
2 hard-boiled eggs*, chopped
1 Tbsp. light mayonnaise (Hellman's® Light is my favorite)
1 stalk celery, finely chopped
1 Tbsp. dill pickle, chopped

Directions: Combine all ingredients and divide in 2 equal portions. Save ½ of the tuna mixture for next day's lunch or snack. Serve on 1 slice of 100% whole wheat or whole grain bread, a bed of fresh spinach, or on a thick slice of tomato. Serve with baby carrots and chunks of cucumber or any other vegetables.

* *See directions for hard-boiled eggs on page 152.*

CHICK PEA AND ASPARAGUS SALAD

Ingredients for 4 servings:

2 Tbsp. olive oil
2 Tbsp. red wine vinegar
3 Tbsp. Parmesan cheese
2 Tbsp. parsley, chopped
Zest of one lemon
¼ tsp. black pepper
2 hard-boiled eggs, diced
½ pound asparagus, lightly steamed, trimmed, and cut into 2-inch pieces
1 15.5 oz. can chickpeas, rinsed and drained
½ cup red onion (if desired)
Bibb lettuce, spinach or romaine (alone or in combination)

Directions: In large bowl, whisk together first 6 ingredients. Add next 4 ingredients and blend well. Divide into 4 servings and place on top of bed of greens.

RAW OR COOKED?

How can you prepare your food to cull the most nutrients from the ingredients? Niche your nutrients and reap the rewards!

GO RAW!

Obtain the biggest health benefits from eating these foods in their natural, uncooked state.

- Beets
- Blueberries
- Chia seeds
- Citrus
- Cocoa
- Coconuts
- Dried Fruits
- Garlic
- Onions
- Red peppers
- Seaweed
- Whole grains
- Nuts *(Soak almonds overnight in water and you will activate their enzymes and enhance their taste. Grind them in a smoothie and bring out more nutrition.)*
- Sprouts and sprouted seeds *(Raw food experts recommend seeking out unpasteurized versions, usually directly from farms.)*

COOK 'EM!

Cooking—often by lightly steaming or sautéing in avocado or olive oil—brings out the best in these colorful (yes, white is a color), nutritious gems..

- Arugula
- Asparagus
- Beans
- Bok choy
- Broccoli
- Brown rice
- Brussels sprouts
- Cabbage
- Carrots
- Cauliflower
- Collard greens
- Kale
- Lentils
- Millet
- Mushrooms
- Oats
- Potatoes
- Quinoa
- Radishes
- Rutabagas
- Squash
- Spinach
- Tomatoes
- Turnips
- Watercress

TOMATO SOUP TOPPED WITH GARLIC CROUTONS

Ingredients for approximately 4 servings:

1 Tbsp. unsalted butter
1 Tbsp. extra virgin olive oil
1 medium onion, chopped
1 stalk celery, chopped
2 cloves garlic, peeled and chopped
1 tsp. fresh parsley, chopped
1 28 oz. can + 1 14 oz. can whole peeled tomatoes with juice
4 cups reduced- or no-sodium chicken broth
Ground pepper to taste
Whole grain, rye, or multi-grain bread, thickly sliced
2 Tbsp. fresh Parmesan

Directions for tomato soup: Heat butter and oil in large pot until it melts. Add onion and celery, stirring until softened (4-6 minutes), then add garlic and parsley. Stir in tomatoes with juice, add broth, and bring to a lively simmer, then reduce heat and cook for 10 minutes, stirring often. When soup has cooled, use a blender or food processor to purée the soup.

Directions for garlic croutons: Toast bread for a few minutes. Peel and cut a garlic clove in half, then scrape on toast and drizzle with olive oil and a sprinkling of fresh Parmesan. Toast again for a few minutes and cut into one-inch squares.

Serving size is one cup of soup with 3-4 cubes of garlic croutons. Serve with salad for a complete meal. Soup may be stored in refrigerator or in airtight containers for up to three months.

BROCCOLI AND CANNELLINI BEAN SOUP

Ingredients for approximately 4 servings:

1 14 oz. can reduced-sodium chicken broth
1 cup water
1 lb. broccoli crowns, trimmed and chopped (about 6 cups)
1 14 oz. can cannellini beans, drained and rinsed
¼ tsp. ground white pepper
½ cup reduced fat shredded extra-sharp cheddar cheese

Directions: Bring broth and water to a boil in a medium saucepan over high heat. Add broccoli, cover and cook until tender, about 8 minutes. Stir in beans, salt and pepper and cook until the beans are heated through, about 1 minute.

Transfer half the mixture to a blender with half the cheese and purée. (Use caution when puréeing hot liquids.) Transfer to a bowl. Repeat with the remaining broccoli mixture and cheese. Serve warm.

Filling up on fiber- and water-rich foods when you begin a meal can help prevent you from overeating later. Research has shown that people who start lunch or dinner with salad or soup end up eating as much as 20% less. Avoid cream-based soups and opt for vegetable varieties.

Molly's Lean & Mean Munchies

To keep your metabolism rate high, it's important to eat at least every four hours. If you're not hungry between meals, simply have a few bites of one of the healthy snack options below.

- 1 cup of unsalted, butter-free popcorn
- 12-14 unsalted almonds, cashews or walnuts (preferably raw)
- Apple with skin or other piece of fruit, rinsed well
- Celery sticks with 1 Tbsp. of peanut butter (limit yourself to 1 serving of peanut butter per day)
- Fiber One®, Luna® or Special K® bar (1 per day). Read labels for fat, sugar, salt, calories and serving size, as some bars are more than one serving.
- No-sugar-added or natural applesauce (no artificial sweeteners permitted)
- Sliced tomato with hard-boiled egg
- 4 whole grain crackers or pita chips with a few tiny chunks of cheese
- Fruit and veggie smoothie if you didn't have one for breakfast
- Leftover vegetables from dinner the previous evening
- Roasted cauliflower and broccoli. Rinse vegetables and cut into small chunks, place in baking pan coated with extra virgin olive oil, toss well and bake at 400º for about 15 minutes or until they begin to brown. Leftovers can be refrigerated for up to 2 days.

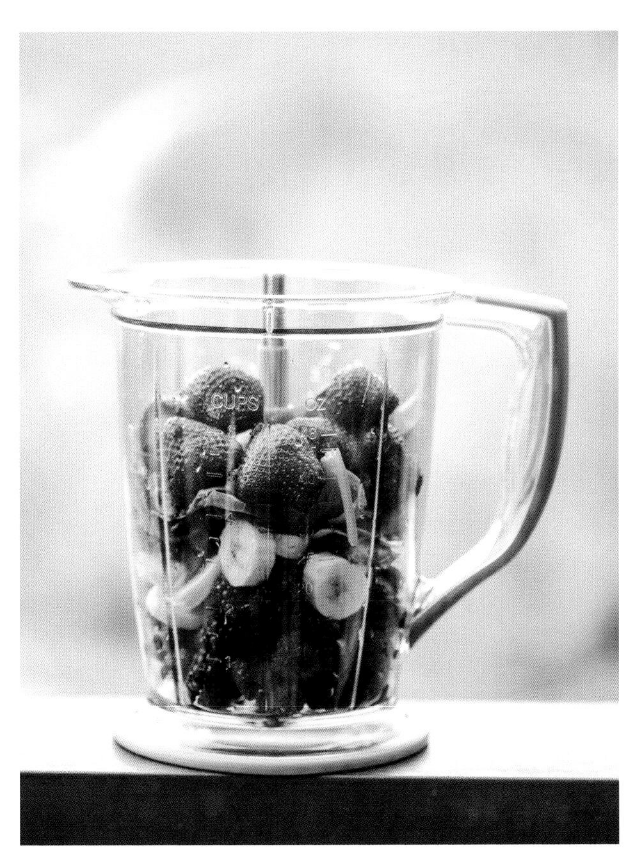

My favorite fruit and veggie smoothie, from start...

...to finish!

Quick, Healthy & Delicious Dinners

Delicious, healthy dinners don't have to be a complicated affair, especially if you keep your kitchen stocked with fresh ingredients and staples from the *Grocery List* (page 82). A number of the recipes here can be done ahead, helping to ensure you round out your day with a nutritious, satisfying meal.

TOMATO, SPINACH AND ARTICHOKE CHICKEN

Ingredients for 4 servings:

2 whole skinless and boneless chicken breasts
1 14.5 oz. can diced tomatoes (with oregano, garlic, jalapeños or other spices added)
1 14 oz. can artichoke hearts, drained, rinsed and broken into pieces
½ bag fresh baby spinach
¾ cup Parmesan or feta cheese crumbles

Directions: Preheat oven to 350°. Rinse lid of can of tomatoes, open and spread 2-3 Tbsp. in a baking dish. Slice chicken breasts at an angle into strips, spread evenly in dish and top with spinach leaves. Pour remaining tomatoes over spinach and top with artichokes. Sprinkle cheese evenly over the mixture and bake for approximately 25 minutes. Check chicken to be sure it is fully cooked. If freezing, bake in foil 9" x 14" pan, cool completely, place wax paper on top of food then cover with plastic wrap and heavy-duty foil to keep in freezer for up to 3 months. Defrost and reheat at 325° until chicken is hot.

Serve this dish with steamed green beans or roasted asparagus. Rinse vegetables thoroughly and break off tips of green beans or ends of asparagus. If roasting asparagus, spray small baking pan with extra virgin olive oil and evenly distribute the fresh vegetables. Drizzle with 1 Tbsp. of extra virgin olive oil and bake at 450° until tender. Use a toaster oven if you have one. (It bakes quicker and uses less energy).

MOLLY'S VEGGIE-LOADED MARINARA SAUCE

I developed this recipe over the years based on a simple marinara sauce. The vegetables enhance the flavor and add loads of vitamins and minerals.

Ingredients to fill 3 32 oz. mason jars:

1 32 oz. can crushed tomatoes
1 cup fresh sweet potatoes, peeled
1 cup fresh butternut squash, peeled
½ cup extra virgin olive oil
5 garlic cloves, minced
½ cup onion, chopped
½ cup celery, chopped
½ cup carrots, chopped
½ cup bell pepper (red, orange, yellow or combination), chopped
2 bay leaves
3 tsp. oregano
3 tsp. basil
3 tsp. thyme
Dash of sea salt
Dash of pepper

Directions: Scrub sweet potatoes, cut into chunks, boil until soft then puree with potato or pastry masher (or use a blender). Do the same with the butternut squash. Sauté the garlic, onions, celery, carrots and bell peppers in olive oil until the onions are translucent (about 10 minutes). Add the tomatoes, sweet potatoes, butternut squash, bay leaves, oregano, basil, thyme, salt and pepper. Simmer uncovered, stirring occasionally, over low heat until the sauce thickens (about 1 hour). Remove from heat and discard the bay leaves. Cool sauce and puree in food processor or blender. Pour into glass jars. Cover and refrigerate to use within the week or freeze for up to 3 months.

Use this sauce over whole grain pasta, zucchini ribbons, roasted cauliflower or salads. Prepare a plate of fresh spinach with ¼ cup of whole grain pasta, then add sauce on top of it all and sprinkle with fresh Parmesan cheese.

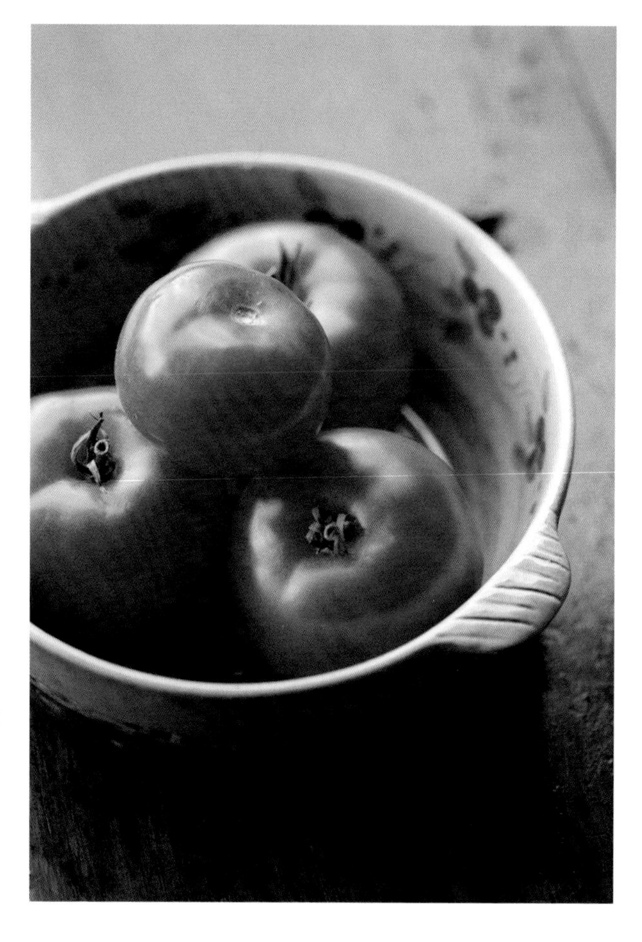

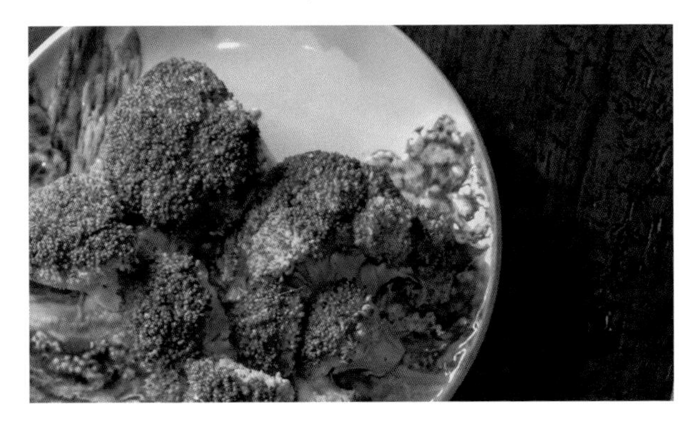

BAKED SALMON WITH CAULIFLOWER PURÉE AND SPINACH SALAD

Ingredients for 4-5 servings:

1 ½ pounds wild salmon
1 whole lemon, washed and cut in half
1 head fresh cauliflower
1 bag baby spinach
1-2 red and/or yellow peppers
1 8 oz. container goat cheese

Directions for Salmon: Preheat oven to 350° and spray baking dish with olive oil. Rinse salmon then place in baking dish. Prick all over with a fork, squeeze both halves of lemon over salmon and bake for approximately 25 minutes at 350° *or* broil for approximately 8-10 minutes.

Directions for Cauliflower Puree: While salmon is baking, rinse cauliflower, cut in small chunks and steam until soft. Puree in food processor with 1 Tbsp. butter or olive oil and cover with foil to keep warm.

Directions for Spinach Salad: Cut red peppers into bite-size pieces, mix them with spinach and crumble goat cheese on top of salad.

ZESTY SOUTHWESTERN SALAD IN CROCK POT

Ingredients for 5-6 servings:

Whole skinless chicken breasts (4 pieces)
Jar salsa (medium or hot, depending on your taste)
1 can corn
1 can black beans
1 package 2% milk Mexican cheese or reduced-fat cheddar
2 avocados
½ bag fresh baby spinach
2 stalks romaine lettuce

Directions: In the morning, rinse chicken breasts in warm water and shake off excess moisture. Spread 1/3 jar of salsa in crock pot, place chicken on top and spread remaining salsa over chicken. Cook on low setting for at least 6 hours. At dinner time, rinse beans, corn, spinach and romaine, chop lettuce into 1-inch pieces and divide on plates. Mix together corn and beans and warm in microwave or on the stove. Break apart tender chicken with fork and knife and add it with its broth to greens. Spoon corn and beans on chicken, then add sliced avocado. Sprinkle 1 Tbsp. of cheese on top of each portion.

VEGETABLE SOUP

Use a crock pot or large pot on the stove. This is a terrific recipe to make on the weekends and freeze in single-size servings. Eat for lunch or dinner with a salad.

Ingredients for approximately 6 servings:

1 15 oz. can tomatoes (diced and low-sodium)
1 15 oz. can extra-thick and seasoned tomato sauce
2 14 oz. cans low-sodium vegetable or chicken broth
1 16 oz. bag frozen or fresh chopped green beans, thawed
2 cups cabbage, shredded
1 cup potato, cubed
½ cup onion, diced
1 cup celery, chopped
1 green pepper, chopped
2 cups carrots, chopped
2 whole bay leaves
1 tsp. basil
½ tsp. salt
½ tsp. pepper

Directions: In large pot, add tomatoes, sauce, broth, shredded cabbage, potatoes, onion, celery, green pepper, carrots, basil, pepper and bay leaves. Rinse and drain beans, then add to pot and mix well. Heat on medium and simmer for 1 hour, stirring occasionally, until vegetables are tender. If using a crock pot, cook on low for at least 6 hours.

Serve with warm, crusty whole-grain wheat or rye bread. Freeze your leftovers in smaller, reheatable containers for lunch or dinner.

What a blessing it is to have fresh and healthy foods to eat. Double your recipes from time to time and take the extra meals to a homeless shelter.

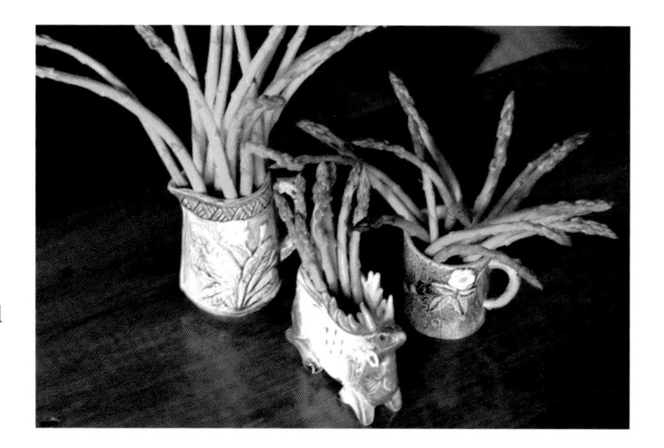

QUICK CHICKEN SPINACH SALAD

Ingredients for 2–3 servings:

2 skinless and boneless chicken breasts (4 pieces)
2 peppers (yellow, green and/or red) and/or lightly steamed broccoli
1 bag baby spinach
½ cup crumbled feta cheese
2 Tbsp. extra virgin olive oil

Directions: Wash and cut chicken breasts into strips. Cut peppers julienne style or trim broccoli and cut into small pieces. Heat skillet with 1 Tbsp. olive oil, add chicken and brown for about 3 minutes per side or until cooked all the way through. Place cooked chicken on paper towels, add more olive oil to pan and sauté peppers and/or broccoli for about 4 minutes. Fill bowls or plates with fresh spinach and add chicken (You will have leftovers to use for lunch or dinner the next day) and veggies. Divide cheese and sprinkle on top.

Serve with ½ cup brown rice or quinoa—½ cup per serving—and additional vegetables.

SLOPPY MOLLYS WITH A VEGGIE TWIST

I created this version of the recipe after trying one from the Deceptively Delicious *cookbook. It's a huge hit with my kids and their friends, and it's loaded with nutrients!*

Ingredients for 6 servings:
½ cup fresh sweet potatoes, peeled
½ cup fresh butternut squash, peeled
1 Tbsp. olive oil
½ cup red onion, chopped
½ cup celery, chopped
2 cloves garlic, minced
½ cup red pepper, chopped in small chunks
1 pound lean ground turkey
½ cup reduced-fat, low-sodium vegetable broth
¼ cup tomato paste
1 Tbsp. Worcestershire sauce
1 tsp. chili powder
Dash of pepper
Whole wheat rolls
½ cup cheddar cheese, shredded
1 avocado, sliced

Directions: Thoroughly rinse the sweet potatoes and squash, cut into 2-inch chunks and boil separately until soft. While potatoes are boiling, sauté onion, celery, red pepper and garlic over medium heat with olive oil until tender. Add the ground turkey breast and continuously break apart with wooden spoon while cooking until meat is no longer pink (about 4 minutes). Stir in vegetable broth. Drain sweet potatoes and butternut squash and puree, then add ½ cup of each to meat mixture. Mix in tomato paste, Worcestershire sauce, chili powder, and a dash of pepper. Cover and simmer until the liquid is reduced (about 10 minutes). Toast whole wheat rolls and spoon mixture on top. Sprinkle with a small amount of cheddar cheese and avocado chunks, if desired. Alternatively, serve open-faced on half of a roll or carb-free over a mix of chopped romaine and spinach.

I serve this with roasted red potatoes cut into chunks, drizzled with olive oil and baked at 400° for 25 minutes until tender and crispy on the outside.

QUICK AND SCRUMPTIOUS MUSTARD CHICKEN WITH ASPARAGUS AND TOMATO

Ingredients for 4 servings:
2 whole skinless and boneless chicken breasts
4–6 Tbsp. Dijon, honey, yellow or any other mustard you desire
2 Tbsp. Parmesan or feta cheese
1 pound fresh asparagus
Two large tomatoes (beefsteak if you can buy at farmers' market)

Directions: Rinse chicken and slice on an angle. Mix a combination of mustards together and spread on chicken. Sprinkle with cheese and bake at 350° for about 25 minutes.

Wash and trim asparagus, brush with olive oil, and place in the baking dish next to chicken for the last 10 minutes of baking. Rinse and slice tomatoes and serve with chicken and asparagus.

ZESTY VEGETABLE LASAGNA

Ingredients for 8-10 servings:

Box of whole grain lasagna noodles
1-2 Tbsp. extra virgin olive oil
1 each red, orange, yellow and green bell peppers, chopped into 1-inch chunks
5 cloves garlic, minced
1 bag fresh baby spinach
2 large eggs
1 15 oz. container reduced-fat ricotta cheese
1 cup fresh Parmesan cheese, plus 2 Tbsp.
1 cup reduced-fat provolone cheese, shredded
1 cup low-fat cottage cheese
1 Tbsp. parsley
1 Tbsp. Italian seasoning
1 Tbsp. basil
1 Tbsp. thyme
¼ tsp. sea salt
1 26 oz. jar marinara or other sauce that has 1.5 grams or less fat and sodium per serving (No more than 10% daily value)

Directions: Preheat oven to 350°. Boil noodles for about 10 minutes in water with a dash of extra virgin olive oil. Drain noodles. Sauté peppers and garlic in olive oil for 7 minutes. Combine eggs, all cheese, spices and salt in a bowl. Spread ¼ cup sauce in bottom of deep, large baking dish (10" x 13"). Place single layer of noodles over sauce, followed by a layer of cheese mixture, then a layer of bell pepper mixture and a layer of fresh spinach. Repeat for 3 more layers, ending with a layer of noodles and sprinkle with fresh Parmesan cheese. Cover with foil and bake for 40 minutes. Remove foil and bake for an additional 15 minutes until

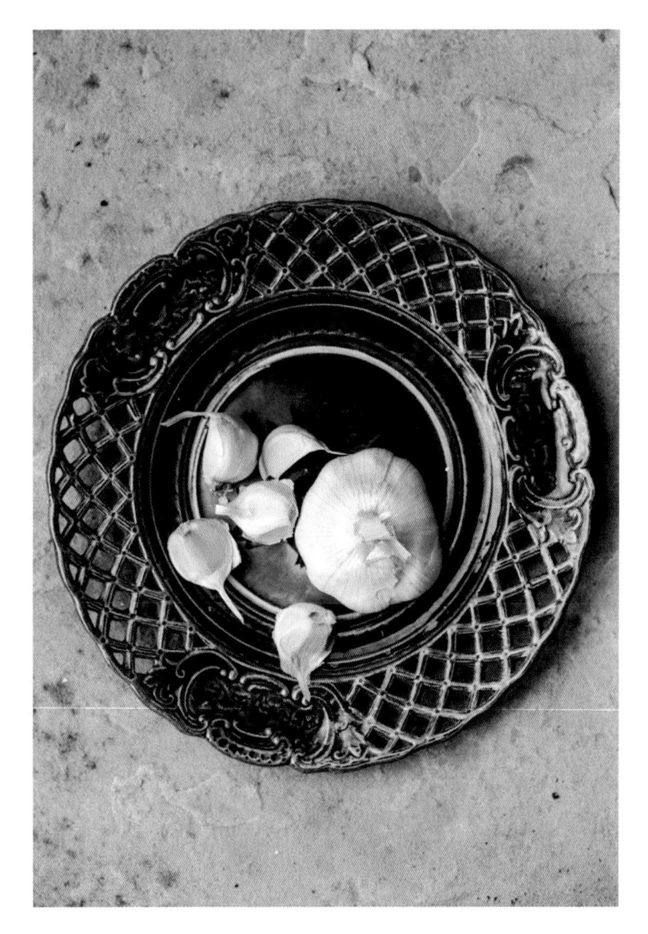

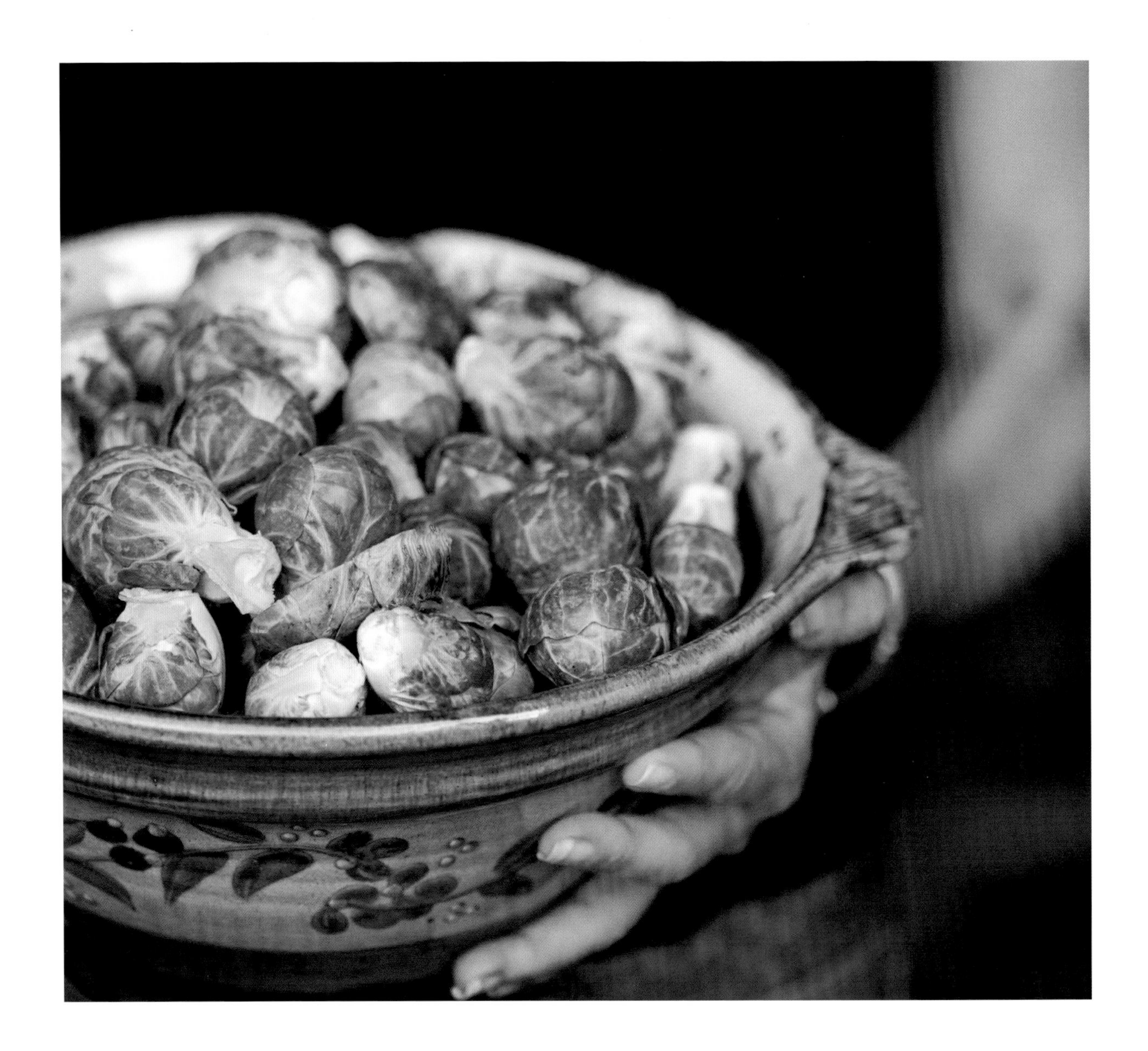

cheese begins to bubble and brown. Cool for at least 20 minutes before cutting.

Serve with fresh green salad of chopped romaine, spinach, avocado and cucumbers tossed with a vinaigrette made of olive oil, red wine, or balsamic vinegar, 1 Tbsp. Dijon mustard and juice from ½ lemon.

ROASTED TURKEY WITH BRUSSELS SPROUTS AND WATERMELON-TOMATO SALAD

Ingredients for 4-6 servings:

Fresh whole turkey breast (5-7 pounds)
1 pound Brussels sprouts
1 whole lemon
2 Tbsp. olive oil
Dash of red wine vinegar
Dash of sea salt
1 Tsp. rosemary, thyme or any other herbs to taste
2 cups watermelon chunks
1 cup tomatoes, chopped
½ cup feta cheese
Dash of pepper

Directions for Turkey Breast: Preheat oven to 350°. Rinse turkey and place in baking dish. Rub 1 Tbsp. olive oil over turkey and sprinkle with 1 tsp. sea salt and herbs. Bake 20 minutes per pound of meat. (For example, if breast is 5 pounds, bake for 1 hour 40 minutes and check that center is cooked.) Remove from oven when fully cooked and let it rest for 10 minutes before slicing. Slice uneaten meat and store in airtight container. Turkey is an incredibly versatile meat. Add it to pasta with vegetables for dinner and use the leftovers for delicious sandwiches the next day.

Directions for Brussels Sprouts: Rinse and cut sprouts in half, steam for 4-6 minutes until tender, add 1 Tbsp. olive oil to skillet on medium high heat, then add sprouts, a dash of sea salt and juice of one lemon. Toss while cooking until lightly browned.

Directions for Watermelon-Tomato Salad: Combine 2 cups of watermelon chunks with 1 cup of tomato chunks, then drizzle with 1-2 Tbsp. olive oil, a dash of red wine vinegar and lemon juice. Sprinkle feta cheese on top.

Sides Without Shame

These side dishes enhance your meals with variety in textures and taste and help you feel satisfied. Limit yourself to a serving size of ½–1 cup.

CUCUMBER, TOMATOES AND AVOCADO

Cut into bite-size chunks and combine. No dressing is needed due to the natural juice from the vegetables and fruit.

BEAN SALAD

Rinse, drain, and mix any combination of beans such as black, cannellini, and chickpeas with 1 chopped red bell pepper, 1 Tbsp. of olive oil, ¼ tsp. of black pepper and 1 Tbsp. fresh dill.

STRAWBERRY FETA SALAD

Slice 1 cup strawberries and combine with 1 Tbsp. crumbled feta or goat cheese and 1 tsp. chopped mint.

BAKED KALE CHIPS

Preheat oven to 350º. Wash and dry one bunch of kale. Tear leaves from stem and place in bowl. Toss in olive oil, a pinch of sea salt and black pepper so that leaves are lightly coated. Place kale on baking sheet in a single layer and bake for 12–14 minutes or until crisp.

MAC & CHEESE MY WAY

Ingredients for approximately 6 ½-cup servings:

2 cups uncooked multigrain elbow macaroni
¾ cup (3 oz) shredded reduced-fat cheddar cheese, shredded
¾ cup (3 oz) Parmesan cheese
½ cup skim milk
2 egg whites, lightly beaten
¼ cup reduced-fat sour cream
1 Tbsp. Dijon mustard
¼ tsp. pepper
1 16 oz. bag frozen petite peas, thawed
1 cup cauliflower, finely chopped
¼ cup soft, whole wheat bread crumbs

Directions: Preheat oven to 350°. Prepare pasta as directed on box, drain well, return to pan and cover. Combine remaining ingredients except for bread crumbs, pour over pasta and stir well. Spread mixture into a 1½ quart casserole dish sprayed with olive oil. Sprinkle bread crumbs on top and bake 30–35 minutes or until golden and bubbly.

CRAZY GOOD GUILTLESS FRENCH FRIES

Ingredients for 4-5 servings:

3-4 whole baking potatoes with skin
2 Tbsp. extra virgin olive oil

Directions: Rinse potatoes and cut lengthwise or into chunks. Drizzle olive oil over potatoes. Bake at 400°, tossing after 10 minutes, until tender and crispy on the outside—about 25 minutes. Serving size is ½ potato per person.

QUINOA AND EDAMAME SALAD

Ingredients for approximately 6 servings:

1 cup uncooked quinoa
2 cups low-sodium vegetable broth
½ cup red bell pepper, chopped and sautéed
2 tomatoes, chopped with seeds removed
2 carrots, peeled, chopped and sautéed
1 small zucchini, cut lengthwise and sliced, with skin on
1 cup frozen edamame, thawed
Zest of 1 large lemon
3 Tbsp. lemon juice
2 Tbsp. extra virgin olive oil
¼ cup fresh leaf parsley, chopped

Directions: Rinse uncooked quinoa and sear in a medium skillet for 5 minutes. Transfer quinoa to a large pot, add vegetable broth and bring to a boil. Cover, reduce heat and cook for 15 minutes or until the water is absorbed and the quinoa is fluffy. Remove from heat and empty into a serving bowl. Add peppers, tomato, carrots, zucchini and edamame, stirring well. Whisk lemon zest, lemon juice and olive oil together, pour over quinoa mixture and toss well. Sprinkle with parsley.

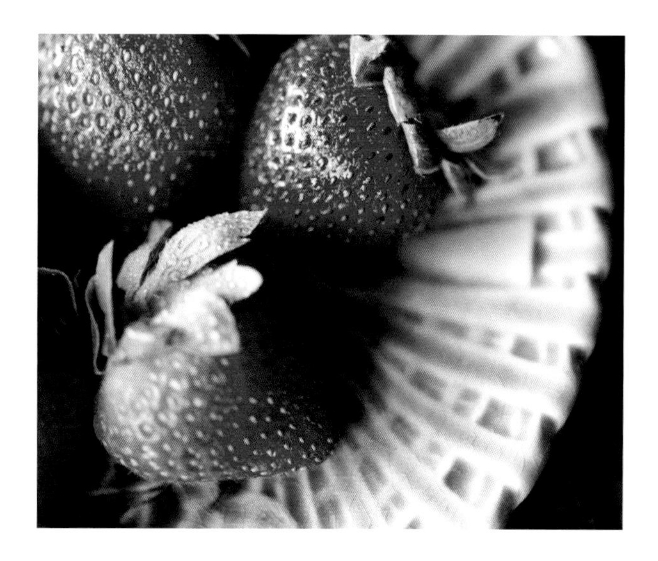

CHERRY TOMATO, BASIL AND FETA CHEESE SALAD

Ingredients for 4-6 servings:

4 cups red and yellow (if available) cherry tomatoes, cut in half lengthwise
½ cup scallions, minced
½ cup fresh basil, thinly sliced
2 Tbsp. extra virgin olive oil
1 Tbsp. balsamic vinegar
¾ cup (about ½ pound) feta cheese, crumbled
Dash of salt
Dash of pepper

Directions: In a small bowl, whisk together olive oil, vinegar, salt and pepper. Combine tomatoes, scallions, and basil in a large bowl, toss with olive oil mixture and top with crumbled cheese.

Weekend Waistline-Friendly Appetizers

Appetizers don't have to be full of empty calories. I've tweaked some popular recipes to create healthier alternatives. The results are so delicious my family prefers them to the high-fat, high-sodium versions.

GUILTLESS GUACAMOLE

Ingredients for 2 cups:
1 zucchini
2 large ripe avocados, skin removed
1 ripe tomato, chopped
¼ cup cilantro
¼ cup chopped onion
2 garlic cloves, minced
2 Tbsp. lime juice
½ tsp. hot sauce

Directions: Dice zucchini and place in glass dish covered with a damp paper towel. Microwave 4-5 minutes or until tender. Drain in a sieve or fine-opening colander and then mash in a bowl with avocado and all other ingredients.

HOMEMADE TORTILLA CHIPS

Ingredients for 32 chips:
8 corn tortillas
Olive oil (in spray bottle)
¼ tsp. sea salt

Directions: Spray both sides of corn tortillas and cut into quarters. Spread on two large baking sheets and sprinkle with a pinch of sea salt. Bake at 375° on the middle and lower racks for 14-18 minutes (or until crisp), rotating the pans from top to bottom and stirring once halfway through to ensure even cooking. These chips also can be served with the *Hummus* and *Southwestern Dip* recipes listed on the following pages.

ANGEL EGGS

Ingredients for 24 halves (serving size is 2–3):
1 dozen hard-boiled eggs*
½ head fresh cauliflower, washed and lightly steamed
2 Tbsp. light mayonnaise
2 Tbsp. Dijon mustard
Dash of paprika

Directions: Cut hard-boiled eggs lengthwise and remove yolks. Add 12 of the ½ yolks to mixing bowl and place the other 12 in refrigerator container to be used at another time. Mash steamed cauliflower and egg yolks together with fork or food processor. Blend in mayonnaise and Dijon mustard, mixing well. Spoon finished mixture into eggs and sprinkle with paprika. Put extra mixture on slices of unpeeled cucumber.

* *See directions for hard-boiled eggs on page 152.*

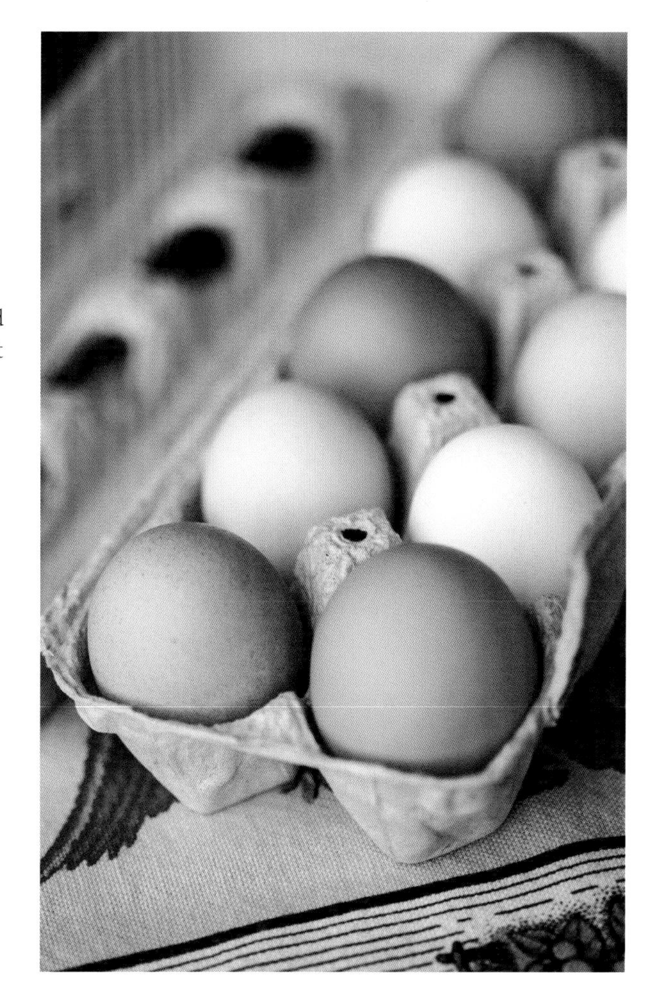

ARTICHOKE HUMMUS

Ingredients for 2 cups or 8 servings:
1 14 oz. can artichoke hearts, drained, rinsed and chopped
1 15 oz. can chickpeas, drained and rinsed
2 Tbsp. tahini or ground sesame seeds
2 Tbsp. fresh lemon juice
1 Tbsp. minced garlic
1 Tbsp. extra virgin olive oil
½ tsp. cumin
½ tsp. hot paprika
1 cup chopped fresh basil

Directions: Combine all ingredients except basil in a food processor and pulse until smooth. Place in bowl and stir in the basil. Serve with fresh vegetables, baked pita chips or homemade tortilla chips.

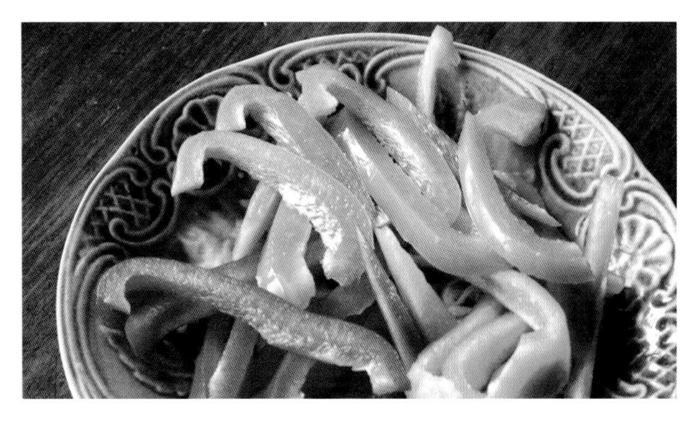

SOUTHWESTERN DIP OR SALAD TOPPER

Ingredients for 6–8 servings as an appetizer or 4 servings as a salad topper:

1 15 oz. can black beans, rinsed and drained
1 14.75 oz. can corn, rinsed and drained, *or* four ears fresh corn, steamed and kernels removed from cob
2 ripe avocados, rinsed, skin removed and cut into medium-sized chunks
1 ripe tomato, rinsed and cut into small chunks with flesh removed
½ cup red diced onion
Juice from fresh lime that has been rinsed and cut in half
1 Tbsp. extra virgin olive oil
1 Tbsp. red wine vinegar
Dash of sea salt

Directions: Combine all items in a large bowl using a soft spatula. Place in festive bowl and keep chilled in refrigerator for up to three hours prior to serving. If you need to make the dip ahead of time, hold off on adding the avocado until serving time so it doesn't turn brown. Serve with homemade tortilla chips, baked pita chips or fresh vegetables.

FABULOUSLY FRESH JULIENNED VEGETABLES

Ingredients:

Asparagus
Bell peppers (red, orange, yellow, green)
Broccoli
Carrots
Celery
Cucumbers
Green beans
Sugar snap peas
(Any seasonal vegetable will work)

Directions: Lightly steam dark green vegetables and rinse in cool water. Cut vegetables julienne style (lengthwise into strips) and display on festive platter. Serve with low-fat ranch dressing.

MOLLY'S OLIVE OIL VINAIGRETTE IDEAS

Making your own dressing only takes a few moments and the result is far healthier than the bottled varieties that are filled with extra fat, chemicals and preservatives. The ratio for preparing a healthy vinaigrette is ⅓ red or white wine vinegar to ⅔ extra virgin olive oil. You can add any herbs you like and, for a richer flavor, add garlic and/or Parmesan cheese.

Dijon Vinaigrette: 1 Tbsp. white wine vinegar, 3 Tbsp. extra virgin olive oil and 1 Tbsp. Dijon mustard.

Herbed Vinaigrette: 1 Tbsp. red wine vinegar, 1 Tbsp. Dijon mustard, 2 Tbsp. parsley and ½ juice from freshly squeezed lemon.

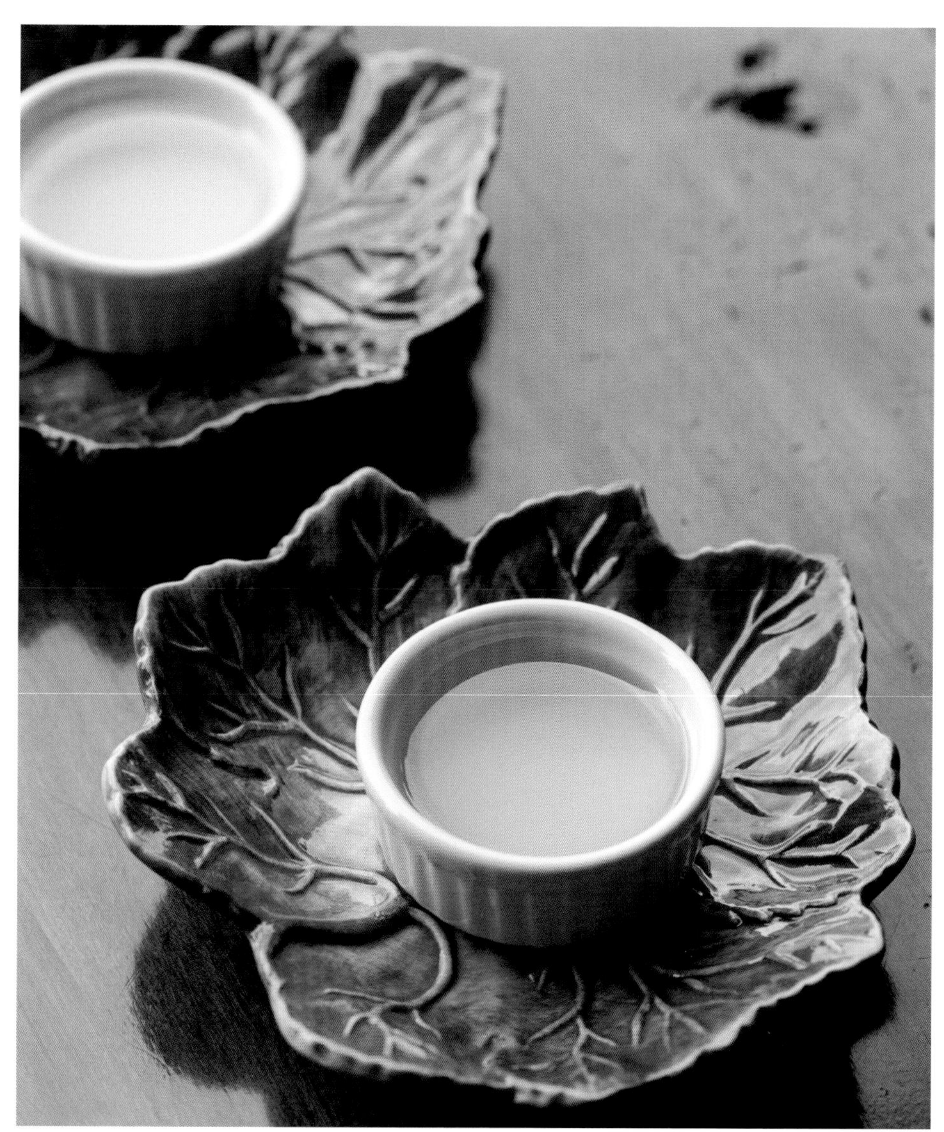

Homemade vinaigrette only takes a few moments to whip up—and it's much healthier than bottled dressings. Use avocado oil or extra virgin olive oil as shown here.

REAL & Figure-Friendly Desserts

Everyone needs a little something sweet from time to time. These wholesome versions of some traditional favorites satisfy the sweetest tooth with healthy ingredients and without harmful chemicals. But limit yourself to the smallest possible serving, and savor every bite.

ALL-BRAN® CHOCOLATE CHIP COOKIES

Freeze the extras so you always have a delicious, healthy treat available.

Ingredients for about 5 dozen cookies:
1 ½ cups sifted all-purpose, non-bleached flour
1 cup sifted whole wheat flour
1 tsp. baking soda
¼ tsp. salt
¾ cup unsalted butter, room temperature
¾ cup sugar
¾ cup dark brown sugar, firmly packed
2 eggs
1 tsp. vanilla
¼ hot water
½ cup All-Bran® (original)
½ cup walnuts, chopped
1 cup semi-sweet chocolate morsels

Directions: Preheat oven to 375°. Stir together dry ingredients and set aside. In large mixing bowl, beat together butter and sugars until light and fluffy. Add eggs and vanilla and beat well. Mix in hot water and then add cereal, flour mixture, walnuts, and chocolate, beating until combined. Place Silpat tray liner on cookie tray. Spoon dough by rounded Tbsp. onto baking sheet (12 per sheet). Bake for 15 minutes or until golden brown. Store in airtight container.

The dough will keep in the refrigerator for up to a week so you can have warm cookies each night. But limit yourself to 2 for dessert.

FORGIVING TREATS:

- 1 Fudgesicle® or 1 cup of sherbet
- 2 small peppermint patties
- 2 oz. dark chocolate (about the size of a credit card) dipped in peanut butter for an extra kick!
- 1 cup frozen grapes, peaches, or berries

BLUEBERRY OATMEAL COOKIES

Ingredients for approximately 24 cookies:

1 stick unsalted butter, room temperature
¾ cup dark brown sugar, firmly packed
½ cup granulated sugar
2 eggs
1 tsp. vanilla
1 ½ cups all-purpose or whole wheat flour
1 tsp. baking soda
1 tsp. ground cinnamon
3 cups Old Fashioned Quaker® Oats (my grandfather's favorite breakfast!)
1 cup fresh blueberries (or from the freezer if you picked them in the summer and froze them like we did)

Directions: Preheat oven to 350°. In large mixing bowl, combine butter and sugars with mixer on medium speed until creamy; add eggs and vanilla and beat until well blended. Add flour, baking soda, cinnamon, and salt and mix well, then mix in oats. With soft spatula, gently fold in blueberries. Spoon dough by rounded Tbsp. (12 per sheet) onto ungreased stainless steel baking sheet (I like stainless steel the best because it bakes cookies evenly). Bake for 10 minutes or until light brown. Cool 1 minute on cookie sheet then remove to cooling rack.

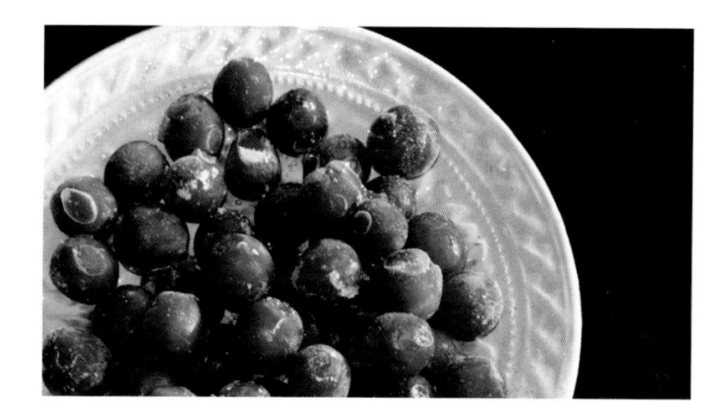

BERRY CRISP

Ingredients for 4 servings:
3 cups fresh blueberries
6 Tbsp. brown sugar
Zest of ½ small orange
¾ cup quick-cooking oats
2 Tbsp. whole wheat flour
⅛ teaspoon apple pie spice, cinnamon or nutmeg
Dash of salt
2 tablespoons cold butter, cut into pea-sized pieces

Directions: Preheat oven to 375°. Place blueberries in a large bowl. If they were just washed, leave them a little wet. If they are already dry add a teaspoon of water. Add 2 Tbsp. of brown sugar and orange zest and gently mix until berries are coated. (I use my hands for this.) Pour berries into a 9-inch pie plate or 9x13 pan. Wipe out the bowl and use it to combine the oats, flour, remaining 4 Tbsp. of brown sugar, spice, and salt. Incorporate the butter pieces with your hands until you have a coarse, crumbly mixture and then sprinkle it evenly over the blueberries. Bake for about 25 minutes or until blueberries are bubbly and topping is lightly browned and crisp.

SCIENTIFIC RESOURCES

1 Maltz, Maxwell. *Psycho-Cybernetics*. New York: Prentice-Hall, Inc., 1960.

2 U.S. Geological Survey. "Water Properties: The Water in You (Water Science for Schools)." Last modified August 9, 2013. http://ga.water.usgs.gov/edu/propertyyou.html.

3 American Society of Hematology. "Blood Basics." Last modified September 15, 2010. http://www.hematology.org/patients/blood-basics/5222.aspx.

4 McHugh, Julia, Nancy R. Keller, Martin Appalsamy, Steven A. Thomas, Satish R. Raj, André Diedrich, Italio Biaggioni, Jens Jordan, and David Robinson. "Portal Osmopressor Mechanism Linked to Transient Receptor Potential Vanilloid 4 and Blood Pressure Control." *Hypertension* 55 (2010): 1438-1443. doi: 10.1161/HYPERTENSIONAHA.110.151860.

5 Kaplan, A., and I.L. Chaikoff. "The Relation of Glycogen, Fat, and Protein to Water Storage in the Liver." *The Journal of Biological Chemistry* 116 (1936): 663-683.

6 D'Anci, K.E., B.M. Popkin, and I.H. Rosenberg. "Water, Hydration and Health." *Nutrition Reviews* 68, issue 8 (2010): 439-458. doi: 10.1111/j.1753-4887.2010.00304.x.

7 Harpo, Inc. "Dr. Oz's Hydration Handbook." The Dr. Oz Show. Posted online September 20, 2010. http://www.doctoroz.com/videos/dr-ozs-hydration-handbook.

8 Virginia Polytechnic and State University. "Clinical Trial Confirms Effectiveness of Simple Appetite Control Method." American Chemical Society. Last modified September 20, 2012. http://www.vtnews.vt.edu/articles/2010/08/082310-cals-davy.html.

9 Weight Watchers International, Inc. "Water and Health." The Weight Watchers Research Department. Last modified December 17, 2011. http://www.weightwatchers.com/util/art/index_art.aspx?tabnum=1&art_id=56961&sc=808.

10 Harpo, Inc. "How Much Water Do You Really Need?" Leigh Vinocur, MD, FACEP. Last modified November 14, 2011. http://www.doctoroz.com/blog/leigh-vinocur-md-facep/how-much-water-do-you-really-need.

11 Goodman, A.B., B. Sherry, S. Park, L. Nebeling, and A.L. Yaroch. "Behaviors and Attitudes Associated With Low Drinking Water Intake Among U.S. Adults, Food Attitudes and Behaviors Survey, 2007." *Preventing Chronic Disease* 10 (2013): 120248. doi: 10.5888/pcd10.120248.

12 Pepino, M. Yanina, Courtney D. Tiemann, Bruce W. Patterson, Burton M. Wice, and Samuel Klein. "Sucralose Affects Glycemic and Hormonal Responses to an Oral Glucose Load." *Diabetes Care* 36, no. 9 (2013): 2530-2535. doi: 10.2337/dc12-2221.

13 Tellez, Luis A., Xueying Ren, Wenfei Han, Sara Medina, Jozelia Ferreira, Catherine Yeckel, and Ivan E. de Araujo. "Glucose Utilization Rates Regulate Intake Levels of Artificial Sweeteners." *The Journal of Physiology*. Published online before print September 23, 2013. doi: 10.1113/jphysiol.2013.263103.

14 Wansink, Brian. *Mindless Eating: Why We Eat More Than We Think*. New York: Bantam Publishing, 2006.

15 Yuan, Gao-feng, Bo Sun, Jing Yuan, and Qiao-mei Wang. "Effects of different cooking methods on health-promoting compounds of broccoli." *Journal of Zhejiang University SCIENCE B* 10, no. 8 (2009): 580-588. doi: 10.1631/jzus.B0920051.

16 Finucane, Mariel M., et al on behalf of the Global Burden of Metabolic Risk Factors of Chronic Disease Collaborating Group. "National, Regional, and Global Trends in Body-Mass Index Since 1980: Systematic Analysis of Health Examination Surveys and Epidemiological Studies with 960 Country-Years and 9.1 Million Participants." *The Lancet* 377, issue 9765 (2011): 557-567. doi: 10.1016/S0140-6736(10)62037-5

17 BBC News. "Eat Less Processed Food, Say Experts." Last modified March 3, 2003. http://news.bbc.co.uk/2/hi/health/2814253.stm.

18 World Health Organization. "Obesity and Overweight." Last modified July 26, 2013. http://www.who.int/mediacentre/factsheets/fs311/en/.

19 Sixwise.com. "All the Health Risks of Processed Foods—In Just a Few Quick, Convenient Bites." Last accessed June 26, 2013. http://www.sixwise.com/newsletters/05/10/19/all-the-health-risks-of-processed-foods----in-just-a-few-quick-convenient-bites.htm.

20 Warner, Melanie. *Pandora's Lunchbox: How Processed Food Took Over the American Meal*. New York: Scribner, 2013.

21 Ibid.

22 Cai, Weijing, Maya Ramdas, Li Zhu, Xue Chen, Gary E. Striker, and Helen Vlassara. "Oral Advanced Glycation Endproducts (AGEs) Promote Insulin Resistance and Diabetes by Depleting the Antioxidant Defenses AGE Receptor-1 and Sirtuin 1." *Proceedings of the National Academy of Sciences of the United States of America* 109, no. 39 (2012): 15888-15893. doi: 10.1073/pnas.1205847109.

23 Oude Griep, Linda M., W.M. Monique Verschuren, Daan Kromhout, Marga C. Ocké, and Johanna M. Geleijnse. "Colors of Fruit and Vegetables and 10-Year Incidence of Stroke." *Stroke* 42, no. 11 (2011): 3190-5. doi: 10.1161/STROKEAHA.110.611152.

24 Aveyard, P., A. Daley, S. Higgs, K. Jolly, A. Lewis, D. Lycett, and E. Robinson. "Eating Attentively: A Systematic Review and Meta-Analysis of the Effect of Food Intake Memory and Awareness on Eating." *American Journal of Clinical Nutrition* 97, no. 4 (2013): 728-742. doi: 10.3945/ ajcn.112.045245.

25 Pollan, Michael. *The Omnivore's Dilemma: A Natural History of Four Meals*. New York: The Penguin Group, 2006.

26 Centers for Disease Control and Prevention. "How Much Physical Activity Do Adults Need?" Last modified December 1, 2011. http://www.cdc.gov/physicalactivity/everyone/guidelines/adults.html.

27 American Heart Association, Inc. "About Cholesterol." Last modified December 10, 2012. http://www.heart.org/HEARTORG/Conditions/Cholesterol/AboutCholesterol/About-Cholesterol_UCM_001220_Article.jsp.

28 U.S. Department of Health and Human Services. "Cell Phones and Cancer Risk." National Cancer Institute at the National Institutes of Health. Last modified June 24, 2013. http://www.cancer.gov/cancertopics/factsheet/Risk/cellphones.

29 Internet Brands, Inc.; FITDAY.com. "Understanding Metabolism: What Determines Your BMR?" Maria Faires, RD. Last accessed July 25, 2013. http://www.fitday.com/fitness-articles/nutrition/understanding-metabolism-what-determines-your-bmr.html.

30 Lemmer, Jeffrey T., Frederick M. Ivey, Alice S. Ryan, Greg F. Martel, Diane E. Hurlbut, Jeffrey E. Metter, James L. Fozard, Jerome L. Fleg, and Ben F. Hurley. "Effect of Strength Training on Resting Metabolic Rate and Physical Activity: Age and Gender Comparisons." *Medicine & Science in Sports & Exercise* 33, no. 4 (2001): 532-41.

31 Gutin, B., and M.J. Kasper. "Can Vigorous Exercise Play a Role in Osteoporosis Prevention? A Review." *Osteoporosis International* 2, issue 2 (1992): 55-69.

32 Weil Lifestyle, LLC. "Natural Cures for Insomnia." DrWeil.com. Last accessed April 13, 2013. http://www.drweil.com/drw/u/ART02037/sleep-aid.

33 Markwald, R.R., E.L. Melanson, M.R. Smith, J. Higgins, L. Perreault, R.H. Eckel, K.P. Wright, Jr. "Impact of Insufficient Sleep on Total Daily Energy Expenditure, Food Intake, and Weight Gain." *Proceedings of the National Academy of Sciences of the United States of America* 110, no. 14 (2013): 5695-700. doi: 10.1073/pnas.1216951110.

34 Harvard University. "Benefits of Exercise - Reduces Stress, Anxiety, and Helps Fight Depression, from Harvard's Men's Health Watch." Harvard Health Publications. Posted online February 2011. http://www.health.harvard.edu/press_releases/benefits-of-exercisereduces-stress-anxiety-and-helps-fight-depression.

35 Hamilton, Lisa Dawn, Emily A. Fogle, and Cindy M. Meston. "The Roles of Testosterone and Alpha-Amylase in Exercise-Induced Sexual Arousal in Women." *The Journal of Sexual Medicine* 5, no. 4 (2008): 845-53. doi: 10.1111/j.1743-6109.2007.00751.x.

36 Heydari, M., J. Freund, and S.H. Boutcher. "The Effect of High-Intensity Intermittent Exercise on Body Composition of Overweight Young Males." Journal of Obesity (2012): article ID 480467, 8 pages. doi: 10.1155/2012/480467.

37 Nerburn, Kent. *Small Graces: The Quiet Gifts of Everyday Life*. Novato, CA: New World Library, 1998.

38 Carnegie Mellon University. "Volunteering Reduces Risk of Hypertension in Older Adults, Carnegie Mellon Research Shows." Shilo Rea. Last modified August 15, 2013. http://www.cmu.edu/news/stories/archives/2013/june/june13_volunteeringhypertension.html.

39 The University of British Columbia. "Doing Good is Good For You: Volunteer Adolescents Enjoy Healthier Hearts." Posted online February 25, 2013. http://www.publicaffairs.ubc.ca/2013/02/25/doing-good-is-good-for-you-volunteer-adolescents-enjoy-healthier-hearts/.

40 Ibid.

41 Borgonovi, F. "Doing Well By Doing Good: The Relationship Between Formal Volunteering and Self-Reported Health and Happiness." *Social Science & Medicine* 66, no. 11 (2008): 2321-34. doi: 10.1016/j.socscimed.2008.01.011.

42 Lourerio, Maria L., Steven T. Yen, and Rodolfo M. Nayga, Jr. "The Effects of Nutritional Labels on Obesity." *Agricultural Economics* 43, issue 3 (2012): 333-342. doi: 10.1111/j.1574-0862.2012.00586.x

43 Flegal, K.M., M.D. Carroll, B.K. Kit, and C.L. Ogden. "Prevalence of Obesity and Trends in the Distribution of Body Mass Index Among U.S. Adults, 1999-2010" *Journal of the American Medical Association* 307, no. 5 (2012): 491-497. doi: 10.1001/jama.2012.39.

44 Purdue University. "Study: Artificial Sweetener May Disrupt Body's Ability to Count Calories." Amy Patterson-Neubert. Last modified May 23, 2011. http://www.purdue.edu/uns/html4ever/2004/040629.Swithers.research.html.

45 Amin, Amr, Alaaeldin A. Hamza, Khuloud Bajbouj, S. Salman Ashraf, and Sayel Daoud. "Saffron: A Potential Candidate for a Novel Anticancer Drug Against Hepatocellular Carcinoma." *Hepatology* 54, no. 3 (2011): 857-867. doi: 10.1002/hep.24433.

46 American Heart Association, Inc. "Physical Activity Improves Quality of Life." Last modified July 24, 2013. http://www.heart.org/HEARTORG/GettingHealthy/PhysicalActivity/StartWalking/Physical-activity-improves-quality-of-life_UCM_307977_Article.jsp.

"Dance as though no one is watching you.
Sing as though no one can hear you.
Love as though you have never been hurt before.
Live as though heaven is on earth."

SOUZA